Postoperative Cardiac Intensive Care

M. V. BRAIMBRIDGE

MA MB BChir(Camb) FRCS(Eng)
Director
Surgical Cytochemistry Section
Rayne Institute; and Consultant
Department of Cardiothoracic Surgery
St Thomas' Hospital
London

with contributions from

M. JONES MD & J. STARK FRCS

Hospital for Sick Children
Great Ormond Street
London

N. M. KATZ MD & L. C. SHEPPARD MD

Department of Surgery
University of Alabama in Birmingham
Alabama, USA

and a Foreword by

JOHN W. KIRKLIN MD

Department of Surgery
University of Alabama in Birmingham
Alabama, USA

THIRD EDITION

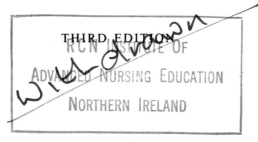

Blackwell Scientific Publications

OXFORD LONDON EDINBURGH
BOSTON MELBOURNE

© 1965, 1972, 1981 by
Blackwell Scientific Publications
Editorial offices;
Osney Mead, Oxford OX2 0EL
8 John Street, London WC1N 2ES
9 Forrest Road, Edinburgh EH1 2QH
52 Beacon Street, Boston
    Massachusetts 02108 USA
99 Barry Street, Carlton
    Victoria 3053, Australia

First published entitled *Post-operative
Cardiac Care* 1965
Second edition 1972
Third edition 1981
Reprinted 1983

Typeset by CCC, printed and bound
in Great Britain by
William Clowes (Beccles) Limited,
Beccles and London

DISTRIBUTORS

USA
    Blackwell Mosby Book Distributors
    11830 Westline Industrial Drive
    St Louis, Missouri 63141

Canada
    Blackwell Mosby Book Distributors
    120 Melford Drive, Scarborough
    Ontario M1B 2X4

Australia
    Blackwell Scientific Book
    Distributors
    214 Berkeley Street, Carlton
    Victoria 3053

British Library
Cataloguing in Publication Data

Braimbridge, M. V.
    Postoperative cardiac intensive
    care.—3rd ed.
    1. Heart-Surgery
    2. Therapeutics, Surgical
    I. Title
    617′.412   RD 598

ISBN 0–632–00233–6

Contents

Foreword

This book on the intensive care of patients early after cardiac surgery by Mr Braimbridge and his colleagues from St Thomas' Hospital in London is an exemplary monograph. In simple terms, Mr Braimbridge details the important aspects of the care of these seriously ill patients. The description in fact is deceptively simple, because its clarity makes it easy to comprehend. What must also be understood is that the execution of the management described must be precisely and skilfully accomplished.

It is because Mr Braimbridge and his superb colleagues use precision and skill as well as knowledge in their intensive care unit that their patients have done well. It is because their approaches have been thoughtful and innovative that they have generated new knowledge which has benefited not only the patients in their unit but patients in similar units all over the world.

This work is recommended for serious study by medical students, house officers, nurses, paramedical persons, and indeed by experienced surgeons. Each group will get something different from the monograph, but each will get something enormously worthwhile.

John W. Kirklin MD

Preface to the Third Edition

Postoperative management after cardiac surgery has undergone marked changes since the first edition of this book. Better understanding of the problems involved, the use of such drugs as potassium, vasodilators, isoprenaline and other inotropes and appreciation of the value of measuring left atrial pressures in left heart disease has made the postoperative management of most patients relatively simple. The advent of cold cardioplegia in particular, with its significantly improved myocardial protection at the time of surgery, has caused a sharp fall in the incidence of postoperative morbidity. But there are still some patients with poor myocardial function in whom the standard of postoperative care makes a critical difference to the prognosis. The third edition of this book is dedicated to the management of these patients with the full programme of assessment and detailed care that is necessary. It is also dedicated to those involved in cardiac surgery for the first time, either those starting a cardiac surgical programme in a new hospital or those who are attached for the first time to an experienced cardiac unit where the problems are fully understood but in which the knowledge is not immediately available to junior staff. The book is not designed for experienced cardiac surgeons to whom the presentation will appear naive.

Dr Branthwaite, who wrote four chapters of the second edition, has been prevented by pressure of work from revising them, but they have been extensively reviewed by my colleagues, Dr Anthony Clement, Dr Robert Linton and Dr Christopher Aps of Department of Anaesthesia at St Thomas' Hospital.

I have been fortunate in having the various chapters revised by specialists in their fields. I am particularly grateful to Dr Tony Wing for revising the chapter on renal failure, to Dr Richard Thompson for that on hepatic failure, to Dr Reginald Kelly for that on cerebral damage, to Professor Wetherley-Mein for the chapter on haematological disorders, to Professor Ilsley Ingram for the section on abnormalities of coagulation, Dr Mark Casewell for the section on infection and Dr David Thompson for the section on hypertension.

Dr Stephen Jenkins from the Department of Clinical Physiology has kindly reviewed the chapter on dysrhythmia. Dr Michael Jones of the

National Institute of Health, Bethesda, Maryland, USA and Mr Jaroslav Stark of the Hospital for Sick Children, Great Ormond Street, London, contributed the chapter on postoperative management of infants after cardiac surgery. Drs Nevin Katz and Louis Sheppard, from the University of Alabama in Birmingham, wrote the chapter on the place of the computer in postoperative cardiac care. I cannot too highly express my appreciation of the time and trouble taken by so many people to improve the calibre of this book. Mrs Diana Hobbs has patiently typed the manuscript and Mr Brandon of the Photographic Department has been responsible for the photographs.

This book could not have been written without the constant help and advice of the sisters and nurses of the intensive therapy unit (Mead Ward) and cardiac surgical unit (Evan Jones and Beatrice Wards) at St Thomas' Hospital. I am especially indebted to Gemma Boase, Julia Chapman, Alice Azzopardi and Clare Meadows, for the sections on immediate measures on return to the ITU and nutrition in particular.

I would particularly like to pay tribute to the work of Dr Ronald Bradley, Consultant in charge of the Department of Clinical Physiology in the Intensive Therapy Unit at St Thomas's Hospital. His application of Sarnoff's concept of changing ventricular function curves to the acutely ill human patient has revolutionized our concepts of postoperative management, particularly of the patient with poor myocardial function. His advice in revision of the chapters on the physiology of the circulation and low cardiac output has been particularly valuable.

Finally, I would like to acknowledge my debt to Dr Frank Gerbode of the Pacific Medical Center, San Francisco and to Dr John Kirklin, now of the Department of Surgery, University of Alabama in Birmingham, USA. My first introduction to effective postoperative cardiac care was while visiting Dr Kirklin at the Mayo Clinic in 1957 and many of the principles established there were applied successfully with Dr Frank Gerbode at Stanford University Hospital in San Francisco and they have remained as essentials of our practice ever since.

CHAPTER 1

The Postoperative
Cardiac Patient

In order to define the problems of postoperative cardiac intensive care, it is necessary to consider what is meant in the present context by the terms cardiac patient, postoperative period and intensive care.

A *cardiac patient* is loosely defined as one who has undergone surgery of the heart or great vessels in the thorax. Such patients differ from each other and from general surgical cases by virtue of the nature and severity of their lesions, the operative techniques used and the involvement of other systems.

The nature of the lesion from which the patient suffers affects postoperative management profoundly. The patient with a simple persistent ductus arteriosus, secundum atrial septal defect or mitral stenosis represents one end of the scale, allowing reasonably confident prediction of a smooth postoperative course, whereas patients who have undergone surgery for multiple valve disease, severely cyanotic Fallot's tetralogy, pulmonary hypertensive left to right shunts or coronary artery bypass procedures in the presence of poor left ventricular function lie at the other end of the scale and require intensive and skilled postoperative management to prevent unnecessary mortality. The severity of the individual lesion will also effect postoperative management, which must be more stormy with pre-existing cardiac failure or a raised pulmonary vascular resistance.

The operative technique used in correction of the cardiac lesion affects the postoperative course to some extent. The patient who has required no artificial means of maintenance of the circulation during operation will usually need less attention than one whose circulation has been interrupted for prolonged periods. The operative technique cannot be divorced from the nature of the lesion however, because the more complicated defect needs more time for its correction and hence more sophisticated methods.

The third characteristic of the cardiac patient is the facility with which other systems are affected by alterations in the cardiovascular state. The function of the brain, lungs, kidneys, liver and other vital organs is dependent on an adequate nutrition and will fail if the blood flow and pressure are compromised.

1

The postoperative period is the continuation and reflection of preoperative and operative management, and may be defined as beginning when the last stitch is placed in the patient's skin. An interim period then follows when he is transferred from the operating table to his bed and escorted to the intensive care unit. This interim period may involve half an hour and is a period when the tension and tedium of the operation are relaxed and the patient may receive somewhat cursory supervision by medically qualified staff. The immediate postoperative period which concerns the greater part of this book is the next 72 hours, as it is during this time that the majority of acute complications occur and during which skilful management can make the difference between success and failure.

The third necessary definition of what constitutes *intensive care of a cardiac patient* during the postoperative period. Care may conveniently be subdivided into basic nursing, accurate assessment of the cardiovascular state of the patient and the prevention and treatment of complications.

The modern scientific and physiological approach to surgery that has made the advances in treatment of cardiac abnormalities possible has also devalued basic nursing, which plays such a large part in maintaining the patient's mental and physical well-being. Simple measures for his comfort can be neglected because of the plethora of scientific commitments thrown on trained intensive care nurses which allows them no time to nurse in the accepted sense. Under basic nursing care can be included the proper preparation of the patient and his relatives for the ordeal ahead and the avoidance of loud, brightly lit conferences at all hours around a conscious patient's bed.

The main theme of this book is that there is no substitute for continuous and accurate assessment of the patient's condition during the initial postoperative period. Deterioration can be insidious and become irreversible if not quickly corrected. In established, experienced cardiac centres with a large number of surgical cases passing through the intensive therapy unit, many of the details of assessment and management can safely be omitted, but in the less experienced unit and in the marginal case, extra care will make the difference between life and death. The degree of intensity of assessment necessary is judged from the preoperative and operative findings and procedure, with a simple regime for straightforward cases but a comprehensive scheme in the difficult case that will place in the hands of the medical staff enough data to enable them to tell at any given time which, if any, of the patient's systems is deteriorating and what is the urgency of treatment.

Prevention of complications is feasible if such a regime of assessment is followed because deterioration is diagnosed early enough for simple measures of correction to be effective. Treatment of complications is also facilitated because they are discovered soon and specific therapy begun.

This book is designed as a practical manual for those new to cardiac surgery and those immediately concerned in postoperative cardiac management—registrars, house officers and intensive care nurses—to aid them in the collection of data, interpretation of findings and management of complications. It has been divided into sections by systems, partly for ease of description and partly because it is a positive help to consider individual systems in turn when simultaneous deterioration of several systems confuses recognition of the primary complication.

Having defined the problem of postoperative cardiac care, and the object of writing this book, it would be wise to define what it is not. It is in no sense designed to supplement books on medical management of cardiac problems. Routine medical treatment and detailed dosages of drugs are omitted except where they form an essential part of postoperative management. References to the literature have also been omitted from the text for ease of reading in such a practical manual and the relevant articles collected at the end of each chapter. The physiological background of each complication is considered in only enough detail to make the clinical presentation clear. Familiarity with thoracotomy management is assumed and no space has been assigned to details of underwater seals, pleural complications and the like.

CHAPTER 2

Immediate Measures on Return to the Intensive Therapy Unit

An intensive therapy unit is an essential part of cardiac surgical management. Whether the unit should be devoted entirely to cardiac surgical patients or be part of the general Intensive Therapy Unit of the hospital is a matter for debate. The latter has the advantage of concentrating expensive equipment and medical and nursing expertise rather than scattering them into coronary care, respiratory, renal dialysis and general intensive therapy areas. It also facilitates the training of nurses and the variety makes the unit more attractive to them, a consideration of importance when shortage of intensive care nurses so often limits cardiac surgical practice. It has the disadvantage that cardiac surgery may at times be curtailed by pressure of work from other specialists.

1. Staff

The nursing staff assigned to an intensive therapy unit need to be trained in the special problems of cardiac surgery. Eight-hour shifts allow the maximum continuity of personal attention for the individual patient and the most rest for the nurses. Each shift has to be under the care of a sister or trained nurse, as considerable scientific and diagnostic responsibility rests on the nursing staff. More junior nurses can then be rotated through the unit from the rest of the hospital for training in postoperative management. Nursing in an intensive care unit can be emotionally wearing, because death is harrowing after the effort that has been expended. The more senior nurses therefore need adequate relief and holidays.

The medically qualified staff also need training, because experience in general surgical postoperative management is little preparation for care of the bad risk cardiac patient. This is true also of junior anaesthetic staff unused to cardiac surgery, who may not appreciate the dangers of hypoxia or the value of positive pressure ventilation before respiratory derangement becomes obvious. Ideally, two housemen should rotate daily so that one is always in the unit if the nurses are to receive adequate support but, failing

4

that, a representative of both surgical and anaesthetic staff should be constantly and quickly available for emergencies.

2. Design of Unit

The design of an intensive therapy unit will depend on the individual hospital, as it is often an adaptation of existing accommodation, but there are certain criteria that are universally applicable. It should be near the operating theatre for the rapid transit of patients and treatment of such complications as haemorrhage and tamponade. A single large room accommodating several beds is preferable to a series of small cubicles, because space is more elastic, one nurse can supervise more than one patient when necessary and operative manoeuvres, such as opening the chest for haemorrhage can be performed without limitation of space. Privacy is best obtained by mobile partitions incorporating shelves and cupboards (Fig. 2.1). A separate area is necessary for patients who become infected and this area is best designed as cubicles.

Ample ancillary space is required for storage, sterilization, simple pathological investigations, accommodation for relatives, kitchen and sluice.

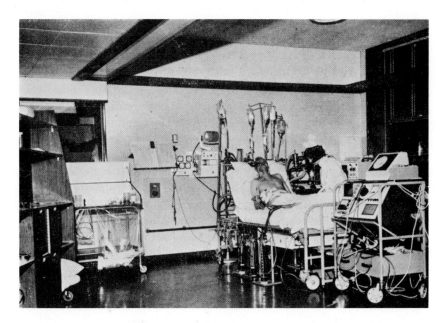

Fig. 2.1. General view of intensive care unit showing (from left to right) mobile shelves, used also as screens, dressing and tracheal suction trolley, chart board, venous and arterial pressures displayed on dials and oscilloscope, patient being artificially ventilated on a Servo ventilator, with chest drainage and calibrated urine bottles on the floor, and emergency trolley with pacemaker, thermometer and electrocardiograph above and cardioscope and DC defibrillator below.

Storage space is needed for bulky equipment such as ventilators, defibrillators and oscilloscopes, and locked cupboards are required for dangerous and other drugs, intravenous fluids, catheters, syringes and sterile packs. Sterilization facilities, such as a ward autoclave, are necessary even if central sterile supplies are provided. A sink suitable for surgical scrubbing is also necessary. A small pathological laboratory is desirable for electrolyte measurement, blood gas analysis equipment, urine testing, microhaematocrit and other simple pathological investigations. Time and staff are not then wasted in sending nurses with samples to laboratories which may be at some distance from the ITU. Relatives, always anxious and sometimes distraught, need comfortable accommodation by day and by night where they can conveniently be seen by the medical staff and from which they can easily visit the patients.

The room itself is painted a restful colour, as the morale of patients and nurses is affected by their surroundings, and walls and floor should permit washing after a septic case, unless enough air changes are ensured by the ventilation equipment. Good lighting includes general lights of adjustable intensity, moveable individual lights over each bed and a powerful shadowless light for emergency operations. Proper ventilation, heating and cooling are desirable.

3. Transfer of the Patient to the Intensive Therapy Unit

The period between closure of the skin incision and stabilization of the patient in the intensive care unit can be a hazardous one. Attention is often relaxed, monitors of the patient's circulatory state are disconnected and the patient is transferred to a bed and then over a varying distance to the care of new personnel relatively unfamiliar with the immediate individual problems.

The principles of management of this period are reduction of movement of the patient to a minimum, continuous assessment of the patient's circulatory state, and efficient transfer of information and immediate policy to the intensive care unit staff. Allowing the patient to resume spontaneous respiration at this time, which may be associated with anxiety, restlessness and hypoxia, can be dangerous in cardiac patients, who are best transferred to the intensive care unit fully anaesthetized if there is any doubt about their circulatory state.

a. REDUCTION OF DISTURBANCE OF THE PATIENT TO A MINIMUM

The intensive care unit bed is brought into the operating theatre to collect the patient, accompanied by intravenous drip poles, clamps for chest drains, hooks for chest drainage, and portable oxygen and nitrous oxide cylinders, anaesthetic bag, catheter mount and CO_2 absorber. The patient is transferred, anaesthetized, directly from the operating table to the bed, ventilated by the anaesthetist from the oxygen and nitrous oxide cylinders, and wheeled quickly to the unit. The patient is accompanied by a member of the operating team who will be able to treat cardiac arrest if it occurs in the corridors.

The regime is relaxed if the patient's condition is good and the operation has not been too severe. The patient is then allowed to breathe spontaneously in the operating theatre and transferred to the intensive care unit with an oxygen mask only.

b. MAINTENANCE OF CARDIOVASCULAR MONITORING

Before the patient is transferred from operating table to bed, electronic monitoring is discontinued. Severe hypotension or cardiac arrest may be precipitated at the moment a critically ill patient is moved and may go unrecognized for an appreciable time unless precautions are taken. The anaesthetist therefore checks the ECG and arterial and venous pressures immediately before disconnecting the pressure lines, and palpates a pulse throughout the period of transfer of the patient from operating table to bed. Electronic monitoring is best reconnected while the patient is being settled in bed in the operating theatre and all the pressures checked to ensure that there has been no deterioration. The venous pressures are raised by transfusion to a level that will allow for bleeding during transfer. The pressure lines are then disconnected, when the pulse again becomes the main monitor during the transfer from theatre to intensive care unit.

A battery operated electrocardiograph and some means of roughly assessing the arterial pressure are invaluable adjuncts during the transfer period. The latter can be as simple as a closed length of air/saline filled tubing connected to the arterial line, so that the anaesthetist can watch the pulse pressure.

c. CONTINUITY OF MANAGEMENT

The nature of the operation, drugs and blood given, general circulatory state, anticipated complications and proposed immediate management can be written on special postoperative forms, or the information transferred to the intensive care unit staff by the anaesthetist and a member of the surgical team. They remain with the patient until monitoring is re-established and the patient's general condition stabilised.

4. Immediate Measures on Return of the Patient to the Intensive Therapy Unit

On return of the patient to the ITU, the most important immediate measures are re-establishment of chest drainage and cardiovascular monitoring. To do this rapidly and efficiently, the area into which the bed will be received is checked by the ITU staff before the patient arrives to ensure that all apparatus is functioning and necessary equipment and drugs are available. The following list includes equipment and drugs that do not necessarily need to be by the bedside but which should be available in the unit.

a. PREPARATION OF BED AREA

All mechanical and electronic apparatus is checked to see that each item is functioning.

(i) MAJOR EQUIPMENT
Such equipment includes:
ECG oscilloscope, ratemeter, leads, plates and electrode jelly, DC defibrillator, leads and electrodes.
Pacemaker.
Electric (or other) thermometer and probes.
Pressure monitoring equipment, already correctly zeroed and calibrated.
Suction apparatus—low volume pumps (Roberts) or low pressure wall suction for chest drainage set to appropriate suction; high volume high pressure pumps or wall suction for aspiration of trachea.
Ventilator, connections, gas supply.

(ii) TRANSFUSION EQUIPMENT
Compatible blood, plasma or plasma substitutes, dextrose 5%, dextrose 4.8% in saline 0.18%, dextrose 50%, normal saline.
Drip sets (adult and paediatric microdrip).
Spring balance (for blood in plastic bags).
Y connections, 3 way taps.
Syringe pump for slow infusion of inotropic or vasodilator drugs.

(iii) CHEST DRAINAGE AND EQUIPMENT
Spare chest drain bottles and connections (in case of breakage).
Artery forceps for occluding tubing.
'Milking' rollers.

(iv) PRESSURE MONITORING EQUIPMENT
Sphygmomanometer and cuff (appropriate size for infant or child): Venous pressure set and scale.
Spirit level.
Connections between transducers and pressure lines.
Flushing fluid (500 u heparin in 500 ml normal saline).

(v) DRUGS
These vary with customs of individual units but include:
Potassium chloride, lignocaine, isoprenaline, dopamine, mannitol, digoxin,

insulin, calcium chloride, adrenaline, Aramine, propranolol, sodium bicarbonate, Nalorphine, Saventrine, morphine, papaveretum, phenoperidine, frusemide, hydrocortisone, protamine, heparin, Rogitine, sodium nitroprusside.
Antibiotics usually used by unit.
Aspirin suppositories.
Warfarin.

(vi) CHARTS, ETC.
Blood and fluid balance charts (Fig. 2.10 and 2.11).
Temperature, pulse, respiration and blood pressure chart. (Fig. 2.9).
Respiratory management chart. (Fig. 2.12).
Request cards and tubes for chemical pathology, haematology and radiographic investigations.

(viii) GENERAL
Reservoir anaesthetic bag and CO_2 absorber for emergency hand ventilation.
Calibrated urine bottle and connection.
24 hour urine save jar.
Nasogastric tube and aspiration syringes.
Mouth and eye toilet trays and saline eye drops.
Adhesive strapping.

b. RECEIVING THE PATIENT IN THE INTENSIVE THERAPY UNIT

When the patient arrives in the ITU, nursing and medical staff reinstitute assessment and management of the patient which has necessarily been reduced in intensity during transfer from the operating theatre. The patient's pulse, arterial and venous pressures are checked, his position is adjusted, ventilation checked, chest drainage tubes connected to suction, urinary catheters and temperature probe connected, blood balance chart begun, the patient sedated if necessary and a clinical baseline then established of the cardiovascular state (Fig. 2.1). Many of these manoeuvres are carried out virtually simultaneously if there are adequate staff present.

(i) POSITION
The patient is initially left lying flat in bed. When his general condition is found to be satisfactory, the shoulders may be raised slightly because pleural and pericardial drainage is more efficient at this angle. The patient is tilted from side to back to other side every 2 hours to prevent basal pulmonary congestion and damage to the skin of the back. The degree of tilt varies with the cardiovascular state and is minimal initially if the circulation is unstable.
   Sitting the patient up rapidly for a chest radiograph at this stage can be fatal, but the radiograph will be of little value if taken supine because a litre

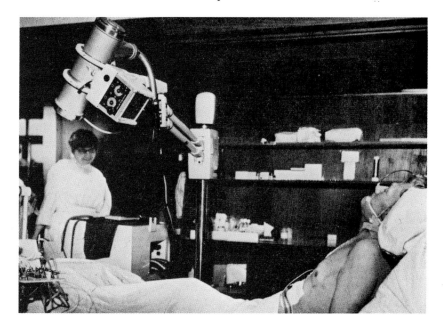

Fig. 2.2. Chest radiography taken at 30° with the minimum of disturbance to the patient.

of blood may lie in the paravertebral gutter without being obvious as more than a general haze. A good compromise is to take the radiograph at 30° (Fig. 2.2).

(ii) VENTILATION

1. *Respiratory rate*
The respiratory rate is recorded whether or not the patient is being artificially ventilated. If he is breathing spontaneously, any movement of the alae nasi or accessory muscles of respiration is reported, as is any tendency to breathe against the machine if he is being artificially ventilated. Both suggest respiratory inadequacy.

2. *Pneumothorax or atelectasis is excluded*
Both sides of the chest are auscultated and the trachea palpated to see that it is central. Chest drains may have been clamped during transit and a pneumothorax or pulmonary collapse may have occurred. These are particularly likely to be missed if they occur on the side opposite to a lateral thoracotomy or if the pleura has not apparently been opened at median sternotomy. A chest radiograph is usefully taken after a few hours as a further check.

3. Oxygen

Oxygen is essential for all cardiac patients in the immediate post-operative period because hypoventilation from the pain of the thoracotomy, sedation, and ventilation/perfusion mismatch from patchy collapse of alveoli tend to produce hypoxia.

If the patient is breathing spontaneously, oxygen is supplied by a face mask or oxygen tent. Neither is entirely satisfactory. Face masks tend to allow a build-up of CO_2 and may not raise the oxygen concentration to 40%. Oxygen tents reach an adequate oxygen concentration even less often because they are continually being opened to attend to the patient and because oxygen tends to leak out round the edges of the tent and through the mattress. In spite of their disadvantages, oxygen masks remain the most practicable way of giving oxygen.

Humidification of the oxygen is important to prevent secretions in the bronchi drying and becoming difficult to cough up or aspirate. Water droplets larger than 8μ do not reach the smaller bronchi and humidification is therefore best carried out with an ultrasonic humidifier or with water vapour at 37°C. Other nebulizers produce droplets that settle in the trachea and main bronchi only, but this may nevertheless be adequate to keep the sputum moist.

4. Artificial ventilation (IPPV)

Intermittent positive pressure ventilation is reasonably continued into the postoperative period in any patient whose circulation is or is likely to become unstable. A ventilator will have been prepared with appropriate connections for an endotracheal tube and checked that it is in working order with all gases flowing correctly. The anaesthetist joins the patient to the ventilator and adjust the rate and minute volume. Subsequent arterial blood gas analysis for Po_2 and Pco_2 check that the settings have been chosen correctly.

(iii) CHEST DRAINAGE

All pleural and pericardial drains are connected to calibrated underwater seal bottles (Fig. 2.3). The tightness of connections and positions of the tubes under water are checked as they may have loosened in transit. The drainage tubes are periodically milked with fingers or rollers to remove clot from the tubes (Fig. 2.4). Some surgeons feel 'milking' is contraindicated after coronary artery surgery.

Suction is applied to obliterate dead space in the chest and so help to reduce haemorrhage. The type of suction used may be low volume with a Roberts type of pump or high volume from wall suction or portable pump. Air bleeds in either type ensure that the negative pressure does not rise above 3 cm Hg. All the drains are connected by Y connections to a single suction source to prevent water being sucked up by one drain, through the chest and down another.

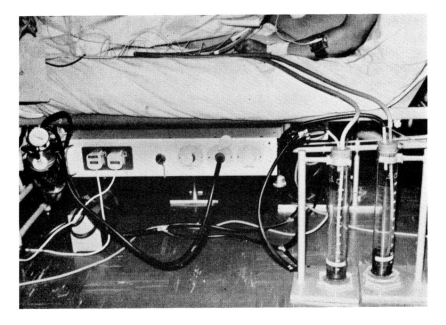

Fig. 2.3. Calibrated underwater seal chest drainage bottles with the level of fluid in them at the time of return to the intensive care unit marked with adhesive tape. A separate bottle is used for each chest drain and all are connected via the air bleed (left) to the same suction source.

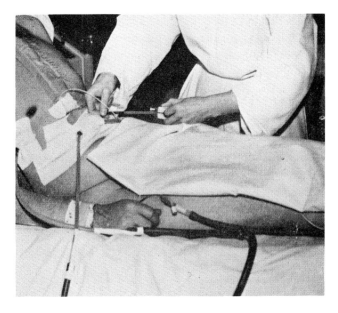

Fig. 2.4. Nurse 'milking' clot from chest drains with rollers.

(iv) OTHER CATHETERS AND CONNECTIONS

1. *Urinary catheter*
The urinary catheter, if inserted, is connected to a calibrated bottle and the urinary output recorded hourly. Urinary tract infection is common after the use of an indwelling catheter and sterility is as necessary in the management of urinary catheters and connections as it is for chest drains.

2. *Nasogastric tube*
A nasogastric tube is not necessary as a routine in adults. Acute dilatation of the stomach is an occasional complication and causes cardiorespiratory embarrassment by pushing up the diaphragm and allowing large volumes of fluid to accumulate in the lumen of the gut. This is particularly true in children. The complication is recognised from the routine chest x-ray showing gas in the stomach.

3. *Temperature*
The temperature may be recorded electrically with a probe inserted into the rectum with which frequent records of temperature can be kept without disturbing the patient. The rectal temperature is 1°C higher than the axillary temperature but is more accurate than the latter if the cardiac output is low, as a patient whose skin is cold due to vasoconstriction may have a high rectal temperature because he is unable to lose heat through the skin.

(v) BLOOD AND FLUID BALANCE
The levels of fluid in the intravenous fluid bottles and chest drainage bottles are marked as soon as the patient reaches the unit (Fig. 2.3). All subsequent measurements of transfusion or drainage are taken from these baselines.

(vi) SEDATION AND ANALGESIA
Adequate sedation is important because pain and anxiety increase the pulse rate, oxygen consumption and cardiac work, and give a tendency to dysrhythmias, including ventricular fibrillation. Oversedation however in a patient breathing spontaneously depresses ventilation and an accurate balance between under- and oversedation is not easy. If the patient is being respired via a nasal or oral endotracheal tube, large doses of sedatives can and should be given to prevent pain and restlessness. Less needs to be given if the patient is breathing spontaneously because the respiratory rate may otherwise be so depressed that ventilation is critically reduced.

The details of sedation in a patient being artificially ventilated are considered fully in Chapter 8. Patients breathing spontaneously are given less sedation. Morphine and papaveretum (Omnopon) are the most effective drugs. They are given intravenously in small doses at a time (Omnopon 2.5–5 mg) rather than large intramuscular injections, because the drug is then immediately effective, however low the cardiac output, its effect wears off fairly rapidly and it can be repeated as often as necessary to maintain the desired level of sedation. It is better to anticipate pain by giving regular small doses, even if the patient is lying quietly, in the early stages because pain, hypertension, oversedation and hypotension cause a see-saw cycle that unnecessarily complicates postoperative management. The use of intrathecal morphine, inserted at the time of induction of anaesthesia, may significantly diminish this demand for analgesia. If pain is not marked, other sedatives may be adequate later.

5. Clinical Assessment of the State of the Patient

Two levels of intensity of assessment of the circulatory state are used after cardiac surgery. A simple regime is adequate following surgery on patients who have undergone relatively minor procedures and who have good myocardial and pulmonary function, particularly in an experienced unit (Fig. 2.13). A more intensive regime is required after operations on patients with poor myocardial or pulmonary function. Analysis of the results of the assessment is considered in detail in Chapter 5.

a. INTENSIVE ASSESSMENT REGIME (FIG. 2.5)

The body reacts to a low cardiac output by restricting the blood flow to less essential areas such as the skin, peripheries and abdominal viscera in order to maintain an adequate blood pressure for perfusion of the brain, heart and kidneys. Clinical evaluation of the state of the circulation therefore entails assessment of the functions of the heart and lungs and the level of perfusion of skin, brain and kidneys.

(i) STATE OF THE MYOCARDIUM
The contractility of the myocardium cannot be easily assessed after cardiac surgery, but a useful indication can be arrived at indirectly by measurement of the venous and arterial pressures, auscultation and the ECG, combined with evidence of adequate perfusion of the skin and other organs.

1. *Venous pressures*
Ideally, both right and left atrial pressures are measured because the filling pressure of each ventricle is critical for its optimal function and each can vary widely independently of the other (p. 39). The right atrial pressure is most easily measured through a catheter passed into the SVC from the jugular vein. The left atrial pressure can be measured through a catheter inserted in the left atrial wall through a purse string suture and brought out through the skin, or indirectly by a Swann-Ganz catheter passed by the anaesthetist before or after surgery to measure pulmonary capillary wedge

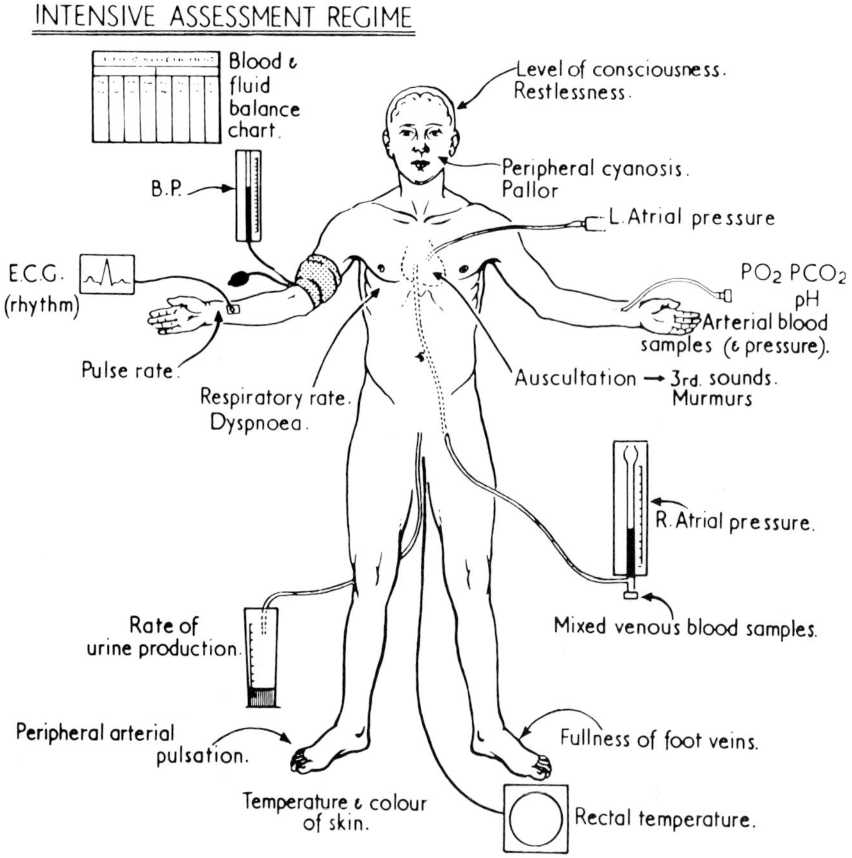

INTENSIVE ASSESSMENT REGIME

Blood & fluid balance chart.

Level of consciousness. Restlessness.

B.P.

Peripheral cyanosis. Pallor

L. Atrial pressure

E.C.G. (rhythm)

PO₂ PCO₂ pH Arterial blood samples (& pressure).

Pulse rate.

Respiratory rate. Dyspnoea.

Auscultation → 3rd. sounds. Murmurs

R. Atrial pressure.

Rate of urine production.

Mixed venous blood samples.

Peripheral arterial pulsation.

Fullness of foot veins.

Temperature & colour of skin.

Rectal temperature.

Fig. 2.5. Diagram of intensive assessment regime showing the various clinical features that are measured and assessed in any patient whose cardiac output is considered to be poor or likely to deteriorate.

pressure. The Swann-Ganz catheter has some associated complications, such as pulmonary haemorrhage.

The pressures are best measured with transducers because the dynamic trace allows the wave form of the venous pulse to be seen. Saline manometers are effective but only give mean pressures (Fig. 2.6). An accurate zero, frequently checked, is required if the pressures are to give infomation of value (Fig. 2.7 and 2.8). This is checked with a spirit level from the sternal angle or left atrial level, depending on the individual unit's practice, every time a pressure is recorded on the chart, because the patient may have moved since the last recording. Drift of the zero in the monitoring apparatus itself is also regularly checked.

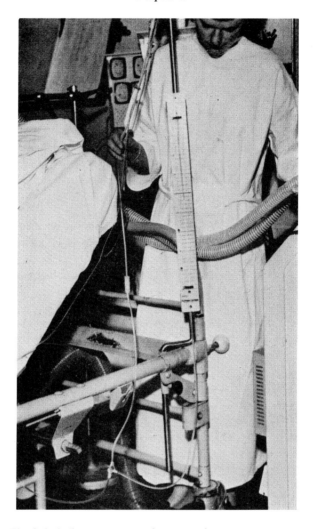

Fig. 2.6. Saline manometer for measuring venous pressure

2. *Blood pressure*

The blood pressure may be measured directly from an arterial line or with a sphygmomanometer cuff. Arterial pressures are best estimated through a catheter left in the radial artery at the time of surgery and connected to a transducer, when the rate of rise of pressure, time to peak pressure and the area under the curve can be directly measured. The catheter can also be used for arterial blood gas sampling. A sphygmomanometer cuff is satisfactory when the blood pressure is reasonably high but tends to become difficult to use when the systolic pressure is below 80 mmHg. An oscillator or Doppler is useful in addition when the blood pressure is low—the systolic pressure is

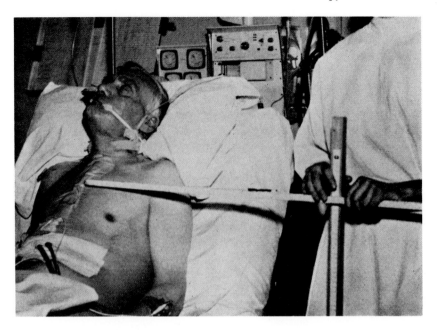

Fig. 2.7. Checking the zero, in this case from the sternal angle, with spirit level and a pole marked with a centimetre scale.

estimated from the sphygmomanometer reading when the pressure or flow is first recorded.

3. *Auscultation of the heart*

The heart is auscultated in every patient. Immediately after cardiac surgery the cardiac output may be low with soft heart sounds and inaudible murmurs and there may be so many pericardial sounds that auscultation is difficult to interpret. A baseline for auscultation is nevertheless valuable. The presence or absence of murmurs is noted. The interval between the aortic second sound and the opening snap of a mitral prosthesis (the isovolumic relaxation interval as the pressure in the left ventricle falls to atrial level) is a useful guide to the left atrial pressure. The presence of a third sound (diastolic gallop) suggests ventricular failure. After operations on the right ventricular outflow tract, the length of the ejection murmur is a measure of the flow through the outflow tract.

4. *Electrocardiogram*

The ECG oscilloscope is connected and the rhythm noted. Loosely applied latex rubber straps and steel plates on all four limbs with frequent changes of electrode jelly may be used (Fig. 2.3) but small, disposable stick-on electrodes are a better and nowadays almost universally adopted alternative.

(ii) PERFUSION OF PERIPHERY

1. *Skin*

The temperature and colour of the skin of the face, knees and feet, and the level on the legs to which warmth extends—the temperature gradient—is noted. Direct monitoring of the temperature of a toe is a valuable measure of peripheral skin perfusion and so, indirectly, of the cardiac output. A temperature probe is strapped to the pulp of the big toe and the temperature recorded with the central temperature. When the two temperatures converge on the chart, the cardiac output is improving. If they diverge—vasoconstriction producing lower skin and higher core temperatures from inability of the patient to lose heat through the skin—the cardiac output is usually falling and this measurement may be the first indication of this happening. Skin temperatures are unreliable in the presence of tricuspid regurgitation which may cause skin dilatation.

2. *Veins*

The fullness and tone of the superficial veins on the dorsum of the feet are noted.

3. *Arterial pulses*

All pulses are palpated—carotid, brachial, radial, femoral, posterior tibial and dorsalis pedis. Systemic embolism causes asymmetrical loss of pulses. In the presence of a low cardiac output and peripheral vasoconstriction, the carotid, femoral and brachial pulses are usually palpable but all distal pulses may be absent.

The pulse rate is recorded. A single rate is recorded if the patient is in sinus rhythm, but both apical and radial rates are separately noted in patients in atrial fibrillation. The pulse deficit—differences between apical and radial rates—records the number of ineffective ventricular contractions.

(iii) STATE OF THE LUNGS

1. *Respiratory rate*

In patients who are breathing spontaneously, fast shallow breathing with moving alae nasi suggests stiff lungs which are often associated with cardiac failure and a raised atrial pressure. The compliance of the lungs is also reduced in pulmonary hypertension. These findings, however, may also be due to atelectasis from bronchi blocked by blood or secretions; which can usually be excluded by auscultation of the lungs or by chest radiography which will show the collapsed areas.

2. *Auscultation of the lungs*

Crepitations at the bases are a sign of pulmonary congestion and oedema. They also occur when a previously collapsed lobe is reexpanding. Râles and

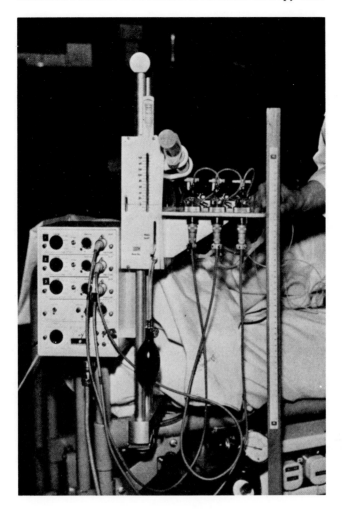

Fig. 2.8. The transducer heads for arterial, left and right atrial pressures are adjusted to the level of the sternal angle.

rhonchi indicate secretions in the bronchi which require physiotherapy or aspiration.

Absent breath sounds over the entire chest suggest a pneumothorax or collapse of the whole lung, both of which can easily be missed unless the lungs are regularly auscultated, particularly when they occur on the side opposite to a lateral thoracotomy. The trachea will deviate towards the side of the pulmonary collapse.

Basal atelectasis causes absent basal breath sounds if the lower lobe bronchus is still blocked, and bronchial breathing if it is patent. Blood or serum in the pleural causes stony dullness on percussion with absent breath sounds and vocal fremitus. Pleural fluid can however be diagnosed unequivocally only by aspiration.

3. *Chest radiography*
A chest radiograph is usefully taken within a few hours of the patient's return from the theatre and again daily until all drains are removed and the circulatory state stabilized. The radiograph may show hilar congestion, pulmonary oedema, atelectasis, pleural fluid, pneumothorax or bronchopneumonia.

(iv) STATE OF THE KIDNEYS

1. *Urine production*
Urine production is measured by inserting a catheter in the bladder and connecting it to a measured container (Fig. 2.1). The volume produced per hour is charted.

2. *Blood and urinary urea*
The level of the blood and urinary urea and a roughly estimated urea clearance are useful indications of renal function. Urinary and blood creatinine and osmolarity are performed if there is any doubt about renal function.

(v) STATE OF THE BRAIN
The level of consciousness, state of the pupils and movement of all four limbs are noted. Lack of response when the anaesthetic is discontinued, particularly if the pupils are asymmetrical and one or more limbs is not moving spontaneously, suggest cerebral damage at the time of surgery and a full neurological examination is performed to establish a baseline for subsequent management (Chapter 11).

(vi) ANALYSIS OF BLOOD SAMPLES

1. *Blood gas analysis*
(a) *Arterial blood.* A cannula left in a radial artery at the time of surgery is the easiest route from which to obtain arterial blood for gas analysis. Arterial puncture is otherwise necessary. Arterial blood is analysed for pH and oxygen and carbon dioxide tensions (Pao_2 and $Paco_2$). Interpretation of the blood gas analysis results is considered in Chapter 7.
(b) *Venous blood.* The oxygen saturation of a mixed venous blood sample is a measure of the cardiac output because, by comparing it with the arterial oxygen sample, an idea can be gained of how much oxygen is being extracted from the tissues. The difficulty of obtaining a true mixed venous sample and the advent of thermodilution cardiac output estimations have made this measurement relatively rarely used however.

2. *Electrolytes*

Sodium and potassium levels are estimated. There is seldom any important change in sodium level immediately after cardiac surgery although the serum sodium may be low initially after haemodilution perfusions. The potassium level may, however, vary widely within a few hours and frequent estimations are necessary until the level remains steady.

3. *Haematological studies*

Knowledge of the packed cell volume (haematocrit) is essential for proper fluid replacement of blood loss. The PCV is ideally kept between 35 and 40%. Clotting studies (Chapter 12) are carried out on any patient who is bleeding excessively.

(vii) CHARTS

A blood and fluid balance chart, a chart showing temperature, pulse rate, respirations, arterial and venous pressures on the same time scale (Fig. 2.9) and, if necessary, a respiratory management chart are started to enable the progress of the circulatory state to be watched.

Blood balance charts keep a running total of all blood lost from each chest drain, the total loss and loss each hour (Fig. 2.10). A simultaneous running total is kept of all blood and other plasma expanders transfused and an hourly balance drawn up. In this way the rate of haemorrhage can be quickly assessed and replacement of overt blood loss assured.

Fluid balance charts keep similar running totals of other fluids infused, urine output and gastric aspirate so that the fluid balance can be assessed at any given moment (Fig. 2.10). A long term fluid balance chart (Fig. 2.11) is used in addition when patients are in the intensive care unit for more than 48 hours.

The volume and type of intravenous fluid replacement for the period up to 8 am the following morning is prescribed so that the appropriate fluid can be started immediately at the correct rate. Allowance is made for infusions of isoprenaline, lignocaine, etc. The volume and type of fluid to be prescribed is considered fully in Chapter 9. 500 ml of 5% dextrose with or without 0.18% saline per square metre of surface area is usually recommended for the day of operation until 8 am the following morning with 800 ml per square metre on the subsequent two days.

Respirator charts are kept for all patients being artificially ventilated (Fig. 2.12). Details recorded include the minute volume, ventilation pressure and checks of routine procedures.

b. SIMPLE REGIME (Fig. 2.13)

The full regime is not necessary after all cardiac surgery and many postoperative courses can be handled on purely clinical evidence. With

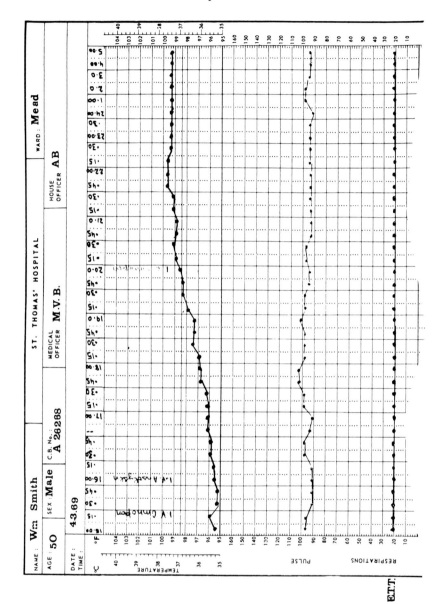

B.T.T.

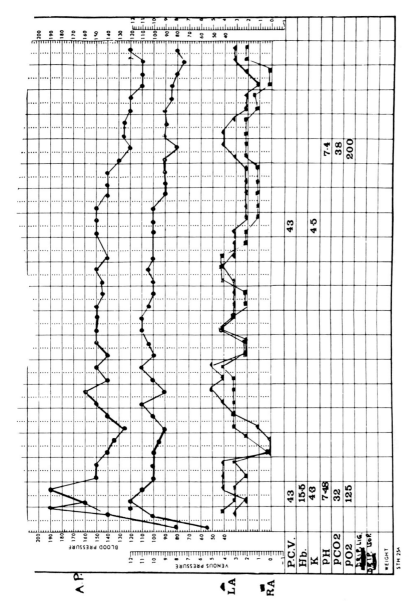

Fig. 2.9. Chart of temperature, pulse rate, respiratory rate, arterial pressure, venous pressures, blood gas and haematological investigations recorded on the same time scale.

ST. THOMAS' HOSPITAL

SHEET NO. 1.

NAME	AGE	WARD	SURFACE AREA	C.B. No.
J. SMITH	40	MEAD	1.68 m²	123456

BLOOD LOSS AT OPERATION 1800 ml.   BLOOD GIVEN AT OPERATION 2,000 ml.

TIME 14/11 DATE	BLOOD BALANCE									FLUID BALANCE							
	Right Drainage	Left Drainage	OTHER	Chemistry	TOTAL	Amount in hour	Blood transfused	Plasma transfused	TOTAL	BALANCE	ORAL	I.V.(1)	I.V.(2)	TOTAL	GAS-TRIC ASPN.	URINE	TOTAL	URINE ml/hr.
1800	0	0		10	10		100		100	+90		0	0	0	0	0	0	
1830	20	10		25	55		300		300	+245		10	5	15	0	10	10	
1900	30	20		25	75	65	540		540	+465		10	10	20	0	30	30	20
2000	140	30		25	195	120	620	120	740	+545		80	40	120	20	70	90	40
2100																		
2200																		
2300																		

Fig. 2.10. Blood and fluid balance chart. The left half of the chart assesses blood balance. The extreme left quarter of the chart consists of columns of running totals of blood loss from each chest drain, blood withdrawn for haematological investigations and the running total of blood lost from the end of surgery until the end of each hour or shorter interval. The next column shows the blood loss during each individual hour. The centre left quarter consists of running totals of blood and plasma expander replacement with a balance estimated at the end of each hour or shorter interval.

The right half of the chart shows the fluid balance. The centre right quarter consists of columns of running totals of oral fluids and fluids other than plasma expanders infused, and the extreme right quarter consists of running totals of gastric aspirate and urine output. The final column shows the urine output in each individual hour.

ST. THOMAS' HOSPITAL

FLUID AND ELECTROLYTE BALANCE CHART

NAME: J. SMITH C.B. No.: 123456 WARD: MEDICAL OFFICER: MEAD HOUSE OFFICER:

SEPT DATE 8 a.m to 8 am	FLUID INTAKE				FLUID OUTPUT			BALANCE	SERUM ELECTROLYTES, ETC.				Hb%	P.C.V.	BODY WEIGHT Kg.	TOTAL INTAKE		URINE ELECTROLYTES ETC.						
	ORAL	5% Dextrose Saline	OTHER	TOTAL	URINE	OTHER	TOTAL		Na mEq/l	K mEq/l	Urea mg/100ml	Bicarb mEq/l				K	Na	Volume ml.	URINE Na mEq/l	Na mEq/day	URINE K mEq/l	K mEq/day	UREA gm/day	SPEC. GRAV.
14/15	0	600	70	670	550	0	550	+120	134	5.2	48	20	15.4	47	68	37	0	550	11	6	69	36	11.2	1010	BLOOD + Protein Trace
15/16	0	1300	50	1350	1600	440	2040	− 690	132	4.8	61	24	15.6	48	(1.7 m²)	50	0	1600	6	9	62	97	11.4	1020	PROTEIN + SUGAR 0
16/17	0	1300	20	1320	980	280	1260	+ 60	130	4.8	54	23	14.0	43		30	0	980	2	2	70	68	12.1	1020	PROTEIN 0
17/18																								

Fig. 2.11. Long term fluid balance chart. Daily totals of fluid intake and output are shown in the left third of the chart with a daily fluid balance. Daily serum electrolytes, electrolyte intake, PCV and urinary electrolytes and urea values are shown on the right.

SURNAME ...SMITH... FIRST NAME ...JOHN...

C B NUMBER ...123456...

DATE ...14.11.70... TYPE OF RESPIRATOR ...ENGSTROM...

ST. THOMAS' HOSPITAL
RESPIRATOR CHART

ENDOTRACHEAL TUBE

TIME	1800	1900	2000	2100	2200	2300
SUCTION	+	+	+	+		
EMPTY TUBES	+	+	+	+		
AIR ENTRY R.	+	+	+	+		
AIR ENTRY L.	+	+	+	+		
MINUTE VOLUME	9	9.4	8	8.3		
TIDAL VOLUME		400	400			
AIRWAY PRESSURE +	25	26	28	28		
AIRWAY PRESSURE –	0	0	0	0		
RATE	20	20	20	20		
OXYGEN	3	3	3	3		
AIR	5	5	5	5		
NITROUS OXIDE						
HUMIDIFIER	+	+	+	+		
TRACHEOSTOMY CARE						
TURN	R	L	L	R		
MOUTH	–	–	+	–		
EYES	–	–	+	–		
ECG LEADS	+	–	–	–		

FORM 690

Fig. 2.12. Respirator chart. Volumes etc. measured and procedures performed are recorded as often as necessary.

STANDARD SIMPLE REGIME

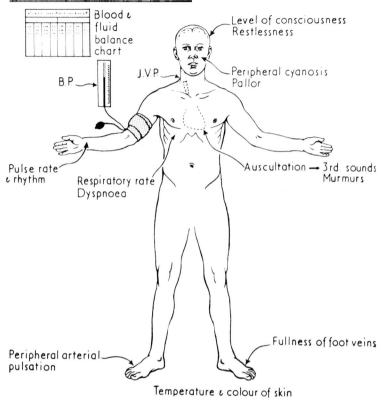

Blood & fluid balance chart

B.P.

J.V.P.

Level of consciousness
Restlessness

Peripheral cyanosis
Pallor

Pulse rate & rhythm

Respiratory rate
Dyspnoea

Auscultation → 3rd sounds
Murmurs

Peripheral arterial pulsation

Fullness of foot veins

Temperature & colour of skin

Fig. 2.13. Diagram of simple assessment regime showing the clinical features that are assessed in patients whose cardiac output gives little cause for anxiety.

increasing experience and volume of work in an established cardiac centre, many of the measures outlined above can be omitted even after major surgery. Such patients are adequately managed without indwelling arterial, venous or urinary catheters. Again, the cerebral state, temperature and colour of the skin, fullness of foot veins and peripheral arterial pulsation, are regularly assessed (Fig. 2.13). The jugular venous pressure with the patient lying at 45° and a sphygmomanometer cuff arterial pressure are adequate measures of venous and arterial pressures.

If unexpected deterioration begins, it is simple to insert a venous catheter via a peripheral vein into the right atrium, pass a urinary catheter, and obtain regular arterial samples by percutaneous arterial puncture or by recannulating the artery. The full intensive regime is thereby reinstituted.

6. Computer Analysis of the Postoperative Course

In some cardiac surgical units, intensive assessment has been undertaken of the value of the computer in postoperative management. The advantages of such a system are that complex variables of the circulatory and respiratory state can be made which may allow an earlier warning of an impending complication than is possible with routine measurements: the information can be relayed to a terminal anywhere in the hospital, including the surgeon's office; medical and nursing staff used to the equipment find it helpful, and the records are useful for research purposes.

The disadvantages are the considerable capital and running costs of the equipment which will be required for several bed stations: the difficulty of ensuring that all the information fed into the computer is accurate: it does not eliminate the need for a nurse by the bedside; and no computer yet made is fully operational 100% of the time.

Randomized studies of patients managed with and without a computer have shown little difference in their eventual clinical outcome. Careful analysis of cost effectiveness of installation of total computerization has resulted in most units around the world, even those with excellent financial resources, deciding to rely on the bedside nurse rather than electronics for routine management. This decision has been reinforced by the marked improvement in recent years in myocardial preservation during surgery which has significantly reduced postoperative problems.

Nevertheless units which have adopted the computer for postoperative management are convinced of its value. One such unit is that headed by Dr John Kirklin of the University of Alabama in Birmingham, which is recognised throughout the world for its application of computer technology in this field. Chapter 3 relates their experience of its use.

CHAPTER 3

The Computer in Cardiac Surgical Postoperative Care

N. M. KATZ & L. C. SHEPPARD

Optimal postoperative care of cardiac surgical patients requires intensive nursing and monitoring for early detection of complications with methods to implement required interventions efficiently and precisely. Although post-operative care may be excellent without the aid of computer technology, the number of highly trained and experienced nurses is limited and an automated system can provide important support for a postoperative care programme. Such a computerized system has been developed by Sheppard and his colleagues and employed in the postoperative management of cardiac surgical patients at the University of Alabama since 1967 (Sheppard *et al* 1968, 1973, 1977, 1979, 1980).

1. Integration of the Computer System into the Postoperative Care Programme

At present two computers are employed in the intensive therapy unit. Of the 14 beds which are equipped for computer-assisted care, 10 are connected to a Hewlett-Packard 2112 computer and the other 4 connected to a DEC PDP 11/20 which is part of a system designed by Roche Medical Electronics. Computer terminals with entry keyboards and video displays are located between each pair of beds. An additional terminal is situated in the nearby laboratory for manual entry of clinical test results (Sheppard 1979).

The automated system performs the following tasks:
(a) Measurements of haemodynamic variables, chest tube drainage, urine output and body temperature.
(b) Storage of these measurements and manually entered observations.
(c) Retrieval and video display of data in tabular form with a specified time interval between data points.
(d) Charting of the data in permanent form for patient care records.

(e) Computations for determination of acid-base balance and administration of drug infusions.
(f) Infusion of blood or fluid within limits to maintain a specified preload, as measured by left atrial pressure.
(g) Infusion of antihypertensive agents to maintain afterload below a specified limit as measured by mean systemic arterial pressure.
(h) Storage of preset rules for postoperative management with the capacity to signal specified interventions.

The usefulness of these functions depends on a postoperative management programme based on orderly rules and organized by body systems. The function of each system is analysed and a plan constructed for further data collection and necessary interventions. This method facilitates rapid reviews of a patient's fluctuating clinical state to allow early detection of complications (Kirklin 1970; Katz & Ottinger 1976). Organization structured by systems is particularly appropriate for cardiac surgical patients in that cardiopulmonary bypass affects all body systems to some degree.

Standard protocols of patient care are used wherever feasible. Such protocols insure consistent application of scientific knowledge to management and facilitate recognition of abnormal responses to interventions. They are particularly efficient in caring for large numbers of patients.

2. Measurements

At the time of induction of anaesthesia, a plastic cannula is inserted into the radial artery. During the operation, polyvinyl catheters are brought out from the right atrium and left atrium (or pulmonary artery). In the intensive care unit, the physiological signals are converted to electrical waveforms by Statham P231D pressure transducers used with continuous catheter flush systems (Gardner *et al* 1970) and the wave forms are displayed continuously on the nonfade display (monitor). The *systolic, diastolic* and *mean arterial pressures* are determined electronically and displayed digitally. *Mean right and left atrial pressures* are monitored in the same manner. The *electrocardiogram* is obtained from disposable surface electrodes. The wave form appears on the monitor, and *heart rate* is derived from the signal and displayed digitally. On occasion the *atrial electrogram* obtained from temporary atrial pacing electrodes is monitored (Waldo *et al* 1978). *Rectal temperature* is measured with a thermistor probe. *Urine output* and *chest tube drainage* are determined gravimetrically. A new set of measurements is obtained and displayed automatically every 2 minutes.

In selected patients *cardiac output* is measured by the dye dilution or thermodilution techniques. The central computers are used in the dye dilution determinations with a separate cardiac output computer used for the thermodilution method. All values with the time of determination are entered at the bedside terminal for display and storage. *Arterial blood* gas results and laboratory measurements of *plasma potassium concentration, haemoglobin concentration,* and *mixed venous oxygen tension* are entered manually into the system when ordered. The frequency of these laboratory measurements is determined by the patient's course.

3. Storage, Retrieval and Charting of Data

At 5 minute intervals the automatic measurement values are transferred to disc storage. Other data obtained manually or without the aid of the computer system are stored on the disc after verification of the values. The data for a particular patient may then be recalled in tabular form for videodisplay. The period for trend analysis can be varied by selecting a different time interval between the measurements retrieved: for example, the previous hour's events can be scrutinized by selecting data points at 5 minute intervals. The period for the analysis can be extended by selecting data point intervals of 15 minutes, 30 minutes, 1 hour, 2 hours or 4 hours. The analysis is facilitated by display of the pressures, heart rate, chest tube and urine outputs, and temperatures on the same videoframe. The sequence of cardiac output measurements can be retrieved for display on another frame. Similarly, the series of laboratory test results can be consolidated into a single frame display. The data are printed in tabular form when a full page of measurements has accumulated. These records are inserted into the patient's hospital chart so that manual logging becomes unnecessary. Not all clinical measurements have been automated (for example, the ventilator settings) and some manual data recording is required.

4. Computations

The computer is employed directly in cardiac output determinations by dye dilution (Sheppard *et al* 1973). The time course of the dye concentration is sampled, and cardiac output, cardiac index and stroke volume are computed. The computer has also been programmed to calculate base excess and alveolar oxygen partial pressures from arterial blood gas data and the inspired oxygen fraction (Thomas 1972). To facilitate rapid and error-free institution of drug infusions, a computer programme has been designed to calculate drug infusion rate from dosage and concentration. Standard as well as minimum and maximum dosages are displayed to facilitate selection of the appropriate dose according to patient management protocols. The programme can also be employed to determine the exact dose of an agent being administered from its concentration and infusion rate.

5. Computer-assisted Decision Making

The amount of postoperative bleeding is automatically evaluated by the computer. Criteria for reoperation were established several years ago at the

University of Alabama in Birmingham by analysis of the bleeding patterns of a group of adults and children, some of whom required reoperation. When bleeding exceeds the calculated acceptable hourly limits or the total limit, the computer displays the recommendation 'consider reoperation'. The system in similar fashion recommends administration of sodium bicarbonate when important base deficits are present. When the computer calculated base deficit exceeds 3 mmol/l, the total extracellular base deficit is estimated. The computer automatically recommends administration of 50% of the deficit unless P_{CO_2} is greater than 30 mmHg and pH is greater than 7.4.

6. Computer-regulated Interventions

A closed loop feedback system is available to maintain preload (left atrial pressure) at a given level with specified limits for infusion. A computer-controlled infusion pump infuses a 20 ml volume of blood, plasma or albumin every 2 minutes unless the left atrial pressure exceeds the set limit or total volume limits are exceeded. The total volume is limited to prevent over-infusion and is specified both as volume per square metre of body surface area and as a multiple of the cumulative blood loss. Thus, if the total volume of blood infused reaches the specific limit (for example 250 ml/m²) or reaches the set multiple (for example, two) of infused blood to cumulative blood loss, the computer will not initiate the infusion despite a left atrial pressure below the set limit.

A computer-controlled system for the infusion of sodium nitroprusside avoids excessive systemic arterial hypertension in the early postoperative period (Sheppard 1980). The development of the system was stimulated by the frequent difficulty of maintaining stable blood pressure with manual control of the nitroprusside infusion and the excessive time required to monitor blood pressure and adjust the infusion rate. The system was designed with a bias towards minimizing infusion of the vasodilator to avoid periods of hypotension: increases in infusion rate are limited by the system, whereas decreases in infusion rate are not. The infusion rates are increased, decreased or held constant at 1 minute intervals to regulate the pressure at the desired level.

7. Postoperative Management of the Cardiovascular System

With recent advances in anaesthesia, cardiopulmonary bypass technology, and operative techniques, most patients arrive in the intensive care unit with excellent cardiac reserves. In this regard cardioplegic myocardial preservation has had a major impact on postoperative care. Interventions now may be minimized, though close patient monitoring is still necessary to detect deviations from normal so that additional measures can be instituted promptly.

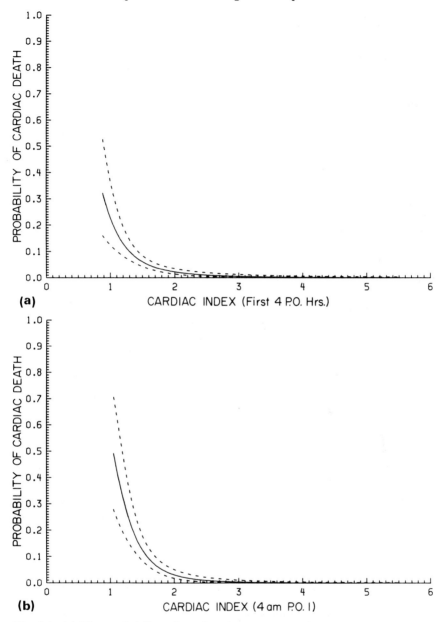

Fig. 3.1. (a) The probability of cardiac death after mitral valve replacement as related to cardiac index measured about 4 hours postoperatively (Conti *et al*). The solid line is the point estimate, and the dotted lines indicate the 70% confidence limits. The risk of cardiac death increases importantly when cardiac index is less than about 1.4 l/min/m^2. (b) At 20–24 hours after mitral valve replacement, the risk of cardiac death is importantly increased when cardiac index is less than about 1.8 l/min/m^2 (Conti *et al*).

Cardiac performance is considered to be adequate if peripheral pulses are palpable, the extremities are warm, systemic arterial pressure is normal or elevated, left atrial pressure is below 18 mmHg measured from midchest level, and urine output is at least 20 ml/hr/m². When all these criteria apply, cardiac index is not monitored, as past experience indicates that it is greater than 2·0 l/min/m². When the adequacy of cardiac performance is in question, cardiac index and mixed venous oxygen tensions are measured serially to determine the need for adjustment of the haemodynamic variables—heart rate, preload, afterload, and contractility. The assessment of cardiac performance is facilitated by calculating a standardized cardiac index for a given preload and afterload as described by Appelbaum and colleagues (1977).

An important relationship between the postoperative cardiac index and the probability of death from cardiac causes can be defined. For example it was found by Conti *et al* that the probability of cardiac death after mitral valve replacement at the University of Alabama in Birmingham increased if the cardiac index in the first postoperative hour was less than 1.4 l/min/m² (Fig. 3.1a). By 20–24 hours after surgery the same curve rose sooner and more steeply as the cardiac index decreased with the risk of cardiac death increasing significantly at a cardiac index of less than 1.8 l/min/m² (Fig. 3.1b.). This relationship was examined in infants and small children also (Parr *et al* 1975), and a similar curve obtained. The risk of cardiac death increased if the postoperative cardiac index was less than 2.2 l/min/m² (Fig. 3.2).

Mixed venous oxygen tension has routinely been measured at the time of cardiac output determinations. This variable, which reflects the oxygen tension at tissue level and therefore the adequacy of the circulatory state, has complemented cardiac output data. Analysis of mixed venous oxygen tension as a determinant of hospital survival in infants and small children (Conti *et al*) indicated that an oxygen tension less than about 25 mmHg is associated with increased risk of cardiac death (Fig. 3.3). Combining measurements of mixed venous oxygen tension with those of cardiac index refines the estimate of cardiac performance (Fig. 3.4).

When the cardiovascular state is unstable (cardiac index less than 1.4–2.2 l/min/m² and mixed venous oxygen tension less than 25–30 mmHg), pacing may be used to increase heart rate to a rate appropriate for age and the computer employed to optimize preload and afterload. In general a left atrial pressure of 14 mmHg, measured from midchest level, is considered optimal, though on occasion it is maintained as high as 18–20 mmHg. Afterload, as measured by mean arterial pressure, is controlled so as not to exceed 10% above the normal value for age. In an adult this implies a *mean arterial pressure limit of about 95 mmHg*. If cardiac performance remains inadequate, inotropic agents are infused at standard rates to increase contractility and consideration given to insertion of an intra-aortic balloon

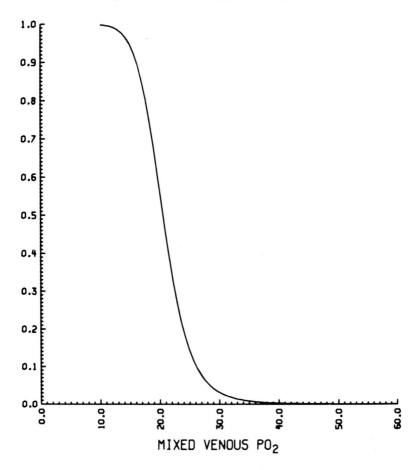

Fig. 3.2. The probability of cardiac death after repair of congenital heart defects in infants and small children as related to mixed venous oxygen tension early postoperatively (Parr *et al* 1975). The risk of cardiac death increases importantly when the value is less than about 25 mmHg.

pump. If practical, each intervention is instituted independently so that its effect on cardiac performance can be clearly defined.

8. Technical Support and Maintenance

A smoothly running computer system requires a skilled supporting staff for sterilizing, calibrating and connecting the system to the patient, maintaining the bioelectric equipment and programming the computer. Well organized routines have been designed for the technical procedures to insure the accuracy of measurements and to facilitate uninterrupted use of the system.

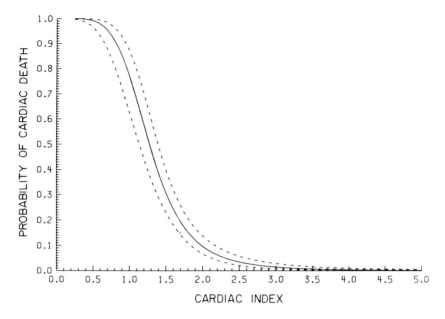

Fig. 3.3. The probability of cardiac death after repair of congenital heart defects in infants and small children as related to cardiac index measured early postoperatively (Parr *et al* 1975). The risk of cardiac death increases importantly when cardiac index is less than about 2.2 l/min/m^2.

At the University of Alabama, failures of the computer system have been few, and problems, when they have arisen, have almost always been with the peripheral units.

9. Effect of the System on Patient Care

The computer system has freed nursing personnel from the routine repetitive tasks of taking and recording measurements and adjusting infusion rates. As a result, nurses have more time for direct patient care: maintaining a clear airway, coaching patients on respirators, supporting the person emotionally, attending to mouth and skin care and observing the patient, which contribute to rapid recovery from cardiac surgery. It has been our experience that with the computer-assisted system of intensive patient care, most patients are sufficiently stable by the morning after surgery to be transferred to semiprivate rooms.

It is at the time that the patient's condition is unstable that the effect of the computer system on patient care is most evident. The increased nursing demands do not compromise the closely spaced accurate measurements

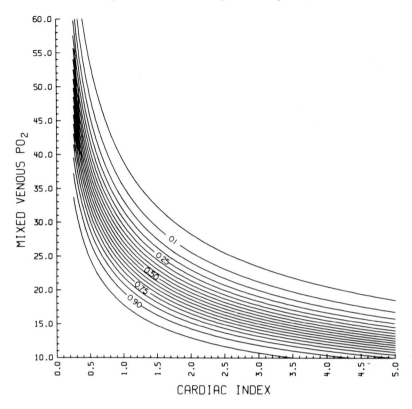

Fig. 3.4. The probability of cardiac death in infants and small children as related to early postoperative mixed venous oxygen tension and cardiac index (Parr *et al* 1975). The contour lines represent the probability of cardiac death.

which are critical in assessing the patient's clinical course. Trends in functions of the various body systems are readily reviewed and physicians can make decisions with organized data. Preload and afterload can be controlled automatically to optimize cardiac performance and infusions can be initiated with minimal chance for error in dose.

In summary, the application of computer technology to cardiac surgical intensive care has provided a high standard of monitoring, independent of differences in nursing training and intensity of patient care required. The computer system has facilitated rapid review of trends in organ function for prompt recognition of complications. Automation has aided in efficient and precise initiation of interventions. Finally the system has freed nursing personnel from time consuming repetitive tasks to allow more intensive direct patient care.

38 *Chapter 3*

REFERENCES

APPELBAUM A., BLACKSTONE E.H., KOUCHOUKOS N.T. & KIRKLIN J.W. (1977) Afterload reduction and cardiac output in infants early after intracardiac surgery. *Am. J. Cardiol.* **39**, 445.

CONTI V.R., WIDEMAN F., BLACKSTONE E.H. & KIRKLIN J.W. Incremental risk factors in primary mitral valve replacement. Unpublished data.

GARDNER R.M., WARNER H.R., TORONTO A.F. & CAISFORD W.D. (1970) Catheter-flush system for continuous monitoring of central arterial pulse waveform. *J. appl. Physiol.* **29**, 911.

KATZ N.M. & OTTINGER L.W. (1976) System-structured management of acutely ill surgical patients. *Arch. Surg.* **111**, 239.

KIRKLIN J.W. (1970) *Systems analysis in surgical patients with particular attention to the cardiac and pulmonary subsystems: 15th Macewen Memorial Lecture.* University of Glasgow Press.

PARR G.V.S., BLACKSTONE E.H., KIRKLIN J.W. (1975) Cardiac performance and mortality early after intracardiac surgery in infants and young children. *Circulation* **51**, 867.

SHEPPARD L.C., KOUCHOUKOS N.T., KURTS M.A. & KIRKLIN J.W. (1968) Automated treatment of critically ill patients following operation. *Ann. Surg.* **168**, 596.

SHEPPARD L.C., KOUCHOUKOS N.T. & KIRKLIN J.W. (1973) The digital computer in surgical intensive care automation. *Computer* **6**, 29.

SHEPPARD L.C. & KOUCHOUKOS N.T. (1977) Automation of measurements and interventions in the systematic care of postoperative cardiac surgical patients. *Med. Instrum.* **11**, 296.

SHEPPARD L.C. (1979) The computer in the care of critically ill patients. *Proceed. IEEE* **67**, 1300.

SHEPPARD L.C. (1980) Computer control of the infusion of vasoactive drugs. *IEEE* (CH 1564-4), 469.

THOMAS L.J. JR. (1972) Algorithms for selected blood acid-base and blood gas calculations. *J. appl. Physiol.* **33**, 154.

WALDO A.L., MACLEAN W.A.H., COOPER T.B., KOUCHOUKOS N.T. & KARP R.B. (1978) Use of temporarily placed epicardial atrial wire electrodes for the diagnosis and treatment of cardiac arrhythmias following open heart surgery. *J. thorac. cardiovasc. Surg.* **76**, 500.

CHAPTER 4

Physiology of the Circulation

The management of circulatory failure is simplified by an understanding of normal cardiovascular physiology and the modifications which are imposed on it by disease. This theoretical background is provided in the present chapter with clinical management being described in Chapter 5.

1. Normal Physiology

The maintenance of aerobic metabolism in the tissues depends on an adequate flow of oxygenated blood through the capillary beds where gaseous exchange occurs. Both total flow (cardiac output) and distribution of this flow may vary according to local requirements and these two aspects are now considered in detail.

a. CONTROL OF CARDIAC OUTPUT

The cardiac ouput is determined by the stroke volume and rate of the heart. The stroke volume depends on ventricular filling and on myocardial contractility. Stroke work (the product of stroke volume and the pressure developed by each ventricle) is a more useful concept than stroke volume alone when considering myocardial function because it takes into account the resistance against which the ventricle contracts.

(i) THE EFFECT OF CHANGES IN FILLING PRESSURE (ALTERING PRELOAD)

It is widely accepted that the Frank–Starling mechanism applies to the intact human heart. In modern terminology, this states that stroke work rises as the end-diastolic fibre length of the ventricle increases. End-diastolic fibre length can rarely be determined in life, and measurements of end-diastolic volume, which reflects fibre length, are difficult. As a result the Starling relationship is often quoted in terms of ventricular end-diastolic pressure. A similar relationship exists between end-diastolic pressure and stroke volume.

In a steady state, the stroke volume ejected by both ventricles must be the same. Any alteration in the stroke volume pumped into the lungs by the right

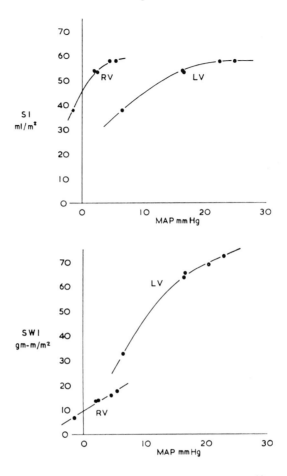

Fig. 4.1. Ventricular function curves from an actual patient for the two sides of the heart. The relationship between (a) stroke index (SI) or (b) stroke work index (SWI) and mean atrial pressure (MAP). RV = right ventricle; LV = left ventricle. (Reproduced from Bradley *et al* 1971, by permission of the Editor, *Cardiovascular Research*.)

heart, produced by changing the right atrial pressure, will briefly upset this equilibrium. If the right atrial pressure is raised, the right heart will pump more blood into the pulmonary circulation than is being removed by the left heart. The pulmonary blood volume will rise until the left heart produces an increase in stroke volume exactly matching that of the right heart. The balance of the system with equalization of the stroke volume ejected by the two sides of the heart is always maintained by small net shifts of blood volume between the systemic and pulmonary circulation.

The function curves showing the relation of right and left atrial pressures to the stroke volume of the normal left and right heart are shown in Fig. 4.1. The relationship between stroke work and end-diastolic pressure may also be expressed graphically, with the function of the two ventricles displayed separately (Fig. 4.1). The filling pressure in the right ventricle is normally a few mmHg lower than that in the left ventricle and the right ventricular stroke work is much less than that of the left because the pulmonary arterial pressure is much lower than aortic pressure.

Clinically, it may be difficult or even dangerous to record ventricular end-diastolic pressure over prolonged periods of time and the mean atrial pressure is often used instead. When the heart is normal, there is a close correlation between mean atrial and ventricular end-diastolic pressures but this is not necessarily true if the heart is abnormal. The relationship between mean atrial pressure and stroke volume or stroke work is then a reflection of the combined performance of atrium and ventricle for each side of the heart.

(ii) THE EFFECT OF MYOCARDIAL CONTRACTILITY
The ventricular function curve may be regarded as an index of myocardial contractility provided that resistance to ejection, heart rate and the degree of inotropic stimulation are constant. If the degree of inotropic stimulation is changed, a whole family of ventricular function curves may be drawn, an upward movement or increase in slope representing improved performance and a downward movement or diminution in slope indicating impaired performance. Such changes may be brought about by autonomic activity or by the action of circulating catecholamines.

(iii) THE EFFECT OF VENOUS TONE AND BLOOD VOLUME
Under normal circumstances, 70–80% of the blood volume is contained in the veins (capacitance vessels, venous reservoir). These vessels are capable of alterations in tone, so that the pressure within them will reflect venous tone as well as vascular volume. Provided the compliance or ease of filling of the ventricles remains constant, an increase in either vascular volume or venous tone will increase the diastolic filling of the ventricle and the stroke volume will rise in accordance with the Starling mechanism.

(iv) THE EFFECT OF ARTERIAL PRESSURE
The normal ventricle can compensate for large changes in resistance to ejection. This adjustment in contractility is an intrinsic property of heart muscle and occurs within a few beats, so enabling a constant stroke volume to be delivered without altering the end-diastolic fibre length.

(v) THE EFFECT OF HEART RATE AND RHYTHM
The normal heart is in sinus rhythm with a co-ordinated contraction of the atria preceding that of the ventricles. In this way atrial systole contributes to

ventricular performance by causing an increase in the ventricular end-diastolic fibre length.

As the heart rate rises, myocardial contractility improves, the proportion of the cardiac cycle occupied by systole decreases and ventricular compliance rises so that diastolic filling and therefore stroke volume are maintained. As a result cardiac output, equal to the product of stroke volume × heart rate, will increase. With extreme tachycardia in normal subjects, the interval for diastolic filling decreases and may be so short that the stroke volume falls.

(vi) CARDIAC RESPONSE TO AN INCREASED METABOLIC DEMAND
Physiological increases in cardiac output are achieved by elevation of the heart rate and an increase in inotropic stimulation of the myocardium. These changes are brought about by activity of the sympathetic nervous system and a rise in the concentration of circulating catecholamines. Although vascular tone in the capacitance vessels increases, so diverting blood towards the heart, the venous pressure does not rise because the ventricles can handle this greater volume by means of improved compliance and contractility, without encroaching on the Starling mechanism.

b. PERIPHERAL DISTRIBUTION OF BLOOD FLOW

Arteriolar resistance, which is dependent on sympathetic tone, is the principal factor controlling the supply of blood to individual organs and tissues, with flow to vital organs such as the heart, brain and kidneys being preserved under all physiological circumstances.

The distribution of flow within each organ is determined by the tone of pre- and post-capillary sphincters, so that blood is directed either through the capillary bed or directly to the venules through the arteriovenous anastomoses. Blood flowing through these latter vessels cannot take part in metabolic exchange. The tone of the pre- and post-capillary sphincters is partly dependent on alterations in sympathetic nervous activity, but is also determined by the concentration of locally produced metabolites. In this way capillary flow can be adjusted to meet the demands of varying metabolic activity in each organ.

The physical behaviour of small vessels is such that widespread closure can occur unless the perfusion pressure exceeds a critical value (the critical closing pressure) but neither perfusion pressure nor total volume flow through the whole organ can ensure that blood is distributed properly to the capillary bed.

2. Modifications Imposed by Disease

Conditions which may adversely affect circulatory performance after cardiac surgery are considered in this section. These include hypovolaemia, loss of vascular tone, pericardial tamponade, myocardial failure and abnormalities in the peripheral distribution of blood flow.

a. HAEMORRHAGE (hypovolaemia)

A healthy adult with a blood volume of approximately 5 litres can sustain the rapid loss of up to 10% of this volume without symptoms or signs of circulatory stress. Sympathetic stimulation causes a progressive increase in venous tone which reduces the capacity of the venous reservoir and enables ventricular filling to be kept constant in spite of a reduced intravascular volume. With further loss from the circulation, changes in venous tone can no longer compensate for the diminishing blood volume. As a result, ventricular filling pressure and consequently the stroke volume tend to fall. The cardiac output and the perfusion of vital organs are maintained by reflex adjustments which include sympathetically-mediated increases in heart rate and myocardial contractility, and constriction of the resistance vessels (arterioles) supplying less vital organs such as the skin, viscera and limb muscles.

With extreme hypovolaemia, these reflexes are unable to maintain either cardiac output or the arterial blood pressure. The perfusion of vital organs diminishes and inadequate coronary flow impairs myocardial performance. In patients breathing air, arterial hypoxaemia results from the mismatch of ventilation and perfusion (Chapter 8), and metabolic acidosis (Chapter 7) develops as anaerobic metabolism occurs in the inadequately perfused tissues.

If recovery occurs without transfusion, the blood volume is initially restored by transfer of extravascular and intracellular water to the vascular space. Subsequently renal retention of salt and water occurs.

b. LOSS OF VASCULAR TONE (vasodilatation)

Resting tone in both the resistance and capacitance vessels is determined by the level of sympathetic stimulation. Certain neurological lesions such as brain stem or high spinal cord injury can reduce or abolish this sympathetic activity, as will a number of drugs which include most general anaesthetics, many sedatives, ganglionic blocking agents and alpha-adrenergic blocking drugs.

Under these circumstances both arteriolar and venous tone are reduced, resulting in hypotension and a low venous pressure. Unless the diminution in either is profound, the stroke volume and cardiac output are often well maintained so that adequate tissue perfusion occurs. However, sympathetically-mediated reflexes which would normally compensate for changes in the circulation are inoperative so that resumption of the upright posture or a small haemorrhage may cause serious hypotension.

C. RESTRICTION OF VENTRICULAR FILLING (tamponade)

A collection of fluid within the pericardial sac will interfere with cardiac filling by obstructing the return of blood from the great veins. The jugular venous pressure is elevated with a sharp descent occurring during ventricular systole when ejection of blood and diminution in cardiac size lower the intrapericardial pressure, and allow blood to flow from the great veins into the right atrium (Fig. 4.2). This systolic descent in the jugular venous pressure tracing may not be seen if heart failure is also present, particularly if there is tricuspid regurgitation.

Pulsus paradoxus, an exaggeration of the fall in systolic and pulse pressure which normally occurs on inspiration, is due in tamponade to a diminution in the effective filling gradient of the left ventricle. As intrathoracic pressure falls during inspiration, the pulmonary venous pressure falls but the intrapericardial pressure is almost unchanged so that the difference between the two is reduced. This inspiratory decrease in filling gradient causes a decrease in stroke volume.

Compensatory reflexes are stimulated by the fall in cardiac output and arterial pressure, and result in tachycardia and peripheral vasoconstriction.

D. MYOCARDIAL FAILURE

(i) IMPAIRED CONTRACTILITY
If the ventricular function curve is used as an index of myocardial contractility, impaired function is reflected in downward displacement and a diminution in slope of the curve (Fig. 4.3) so that eventually both stroke work and stroke volume are virtually independent of changes in filling pressure (Fig. 4.4c).

The possible existence of a descending limb to the curve relating stroke volume to filling pressure deserves mention here. Such a relationship may be demonstrated in the isolated heart so that stroke volume falls as ventricular filling is increased beyond a certain limit. If this were to occur in the intact circulation, a rise in right ventricular end-diastolic pressure would reduce right ventricular stroke volume. This in turn would lower left ventricular end-diastolic pressure and the left ventricle would therefore deliver a larger stroke volume into the systemic circulation. This disparity between right and left ventricular stroke output would eventually displace all the blood from the lungs into the systemic vessels. The demonstration of a slight, apparently negative, slope to the function curve relating stroke volume to mean atrial pressure in certain severely disordered subjects (Fig 4.3) probably represents additional circulatory adjustments such as an alteration in contractility or in the competence of the atrio-ventricular valve.

There are a number of circumstances in which heart failure affects predominantly either the right or the left ventricle and this discrepancy is reflected in the function curves derived for each side of the heart.

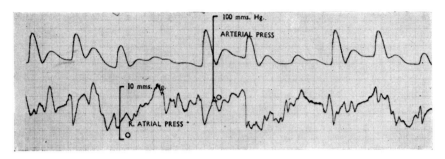

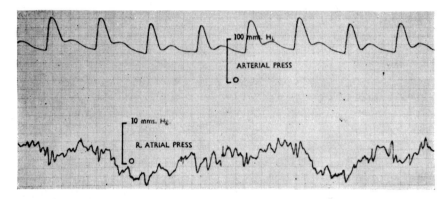

Fig. 4.2. Records of arterial and right atrial pressures in a case of tamponade. (a) Before. (b) After aspiration of 750 ml of blood from the pericardial sac. In (a), there is arterial hypotension and pulsus paradoxus together with a raised right atrial pressure and a dominant systolic descent in the atrial trace. In (b), both pressures are normal.

The curves in Fig. 4.4a were obtained in a man who had recently sustained a myocardial infarction, whereas those in Fig. 4.4b were derived from a patient suffering from pulmonary embolism. In Fig. 4.4a the left ventricular function curve, and in Fig. 4.4b the right ventricular function curve is more depressed and flattened than its fellow when compared with the normal configuration shown in Fig. 4.1. The curves in Fig. 4.4c were obtained in a patient with both myocardial infarction and pulmonary embolism and show extreme impairment of the function of both ventricles.

The clinical importance of these three variants of 'heart failure' lies in the varying ease with which pulmonary oedema may occur. When there is predominant impairment of left ventricular function, high values for the mean left atrial pressure are found while the mean right atrial pressure is not greatly elevated. A slight increase in the mean right atrial pressure will be

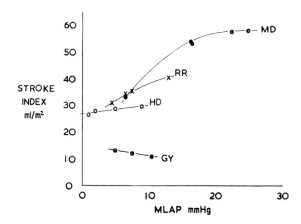

Fig. 4.3. Left ventricular function curves in heart failure.

MD: normal.
RR: following mitral valve replacement; condition satisfactory.
HD: following mitral valve replacement; condition poor.
GY: following mitral valve replacement; condition critical.
MLAP: mean left atrial pressure.

accompanied by a large rise in mean left atrial pressure, and the threshold for pulmonary oedema is reached quickly. If the pulmonary capillary membrane is normal, pulmonary oedema results when the mean left atrial pressure exceeds the osmotic pressure of the plasma proteins (approximately 30 mmHg).

If right ventricular function is more impaired than that of the left, the mean right atrial pressure will exceed the mean left atrial pressure and it is unlikely that the latter will ever reach the level at which pulmonary oedema occurs.

If both ventricles are failing, the mean left atrial pressure may reach the threshold for pulmonary oedema, but the right atrial pressure will also be greatly elevated. The relative function of the two sides of the heart and the risks of developing pulmonary oedema may be inferred therefore by comparing mean right and left atrial pressures.

(ii) DISORDERS OF RATE AND RHYTHM
When the heart is in sinus rhythm, atrial systole augments ventricular filling which would otherwise be achieved solely by passive inflow into the relaxed ventricular chamber. Many disorders of both rhythm and conduction abolish this effect and as a result, the same degree of diastolic filling of the ventricle can only be achieved by an increase in mean atrial pressure. On the left side of the heart this is associated with an increase in pulmonary blood volume

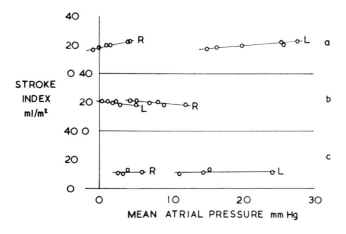

Fig. 4.4. Ventricular function curves.
(a) following myocardial infarction.
(b) following pulmonary embolism.
(c) following myocardial infarction complicated by pulmonary embolism.
In each case, there is impairment of the function of both sides of the heart but in (a) the left ventricle and in (b) the right ventricle is more severely affected.

and a fall in pulmonary compliance so that dyspnoea and orthopnoea may occur.

The heart rate is of particular importance when the stroke volume is low and fixed because it is the only means by which an alteration in cardiac output can be achieved. An increase in rate may then improve cardiac output, but the intrinsic ability to shorten systole and so preserve the diastolic filling interval is impaired in heart failure and if the increase in rate is considerable, the stroke volume and cardiac output may fall.

(iii) HYPERTENSION
The ability to compensate for changes in resistance to ejection without encroaching on the Starling mechanism is limited in heart failure, and a rise in aortic pressure is followed by an increase in left ventricular end-diastolic pressure. If the stroke volume and heart rate remain unchanged, both ventricular stroke work and minute work will increase and the oxygen consumption of the heart will rise. Myocardial ischaemia will result if the coronary blood supply is inadequate to meet this demand.

(iv) RESPONSE OF THE FAILING HEART TO AN INCREASED METABOLIC DEMAND
All the mechanisms which normally increase the cardiac output are less effective when the heart is failing. Tachycardia may already be present and

a further increase in rate may impair diastolic filling of the ventricles. The stroke volume is low and may be dependent on sympathetic stimulation. Both venous tone and venous pressure are elevated at rest and any further rise will cause little increase in stroke volume.

As a result, the cardiac output is unchanged or rises only slightly when the metabolic demand is elevated, for example by restlessness or fever. Selective vasconstriction directs this restricted flow to the heart, brain and exercising muscles while limiting the perfusion of other organs.

e. DISORDERS OF PERIPHERAL PERFUSION

The role of the sympathetic nervous system in modifying the performance of the circulation has been stressed repeatedly. Although sympathetic stimulation tends to maintain the cardiac output, arterial pressure and the supply of blood to vital organs, the distribution of blood within the tissues is altered and this may contribute to circulatory failure by preventing capillary perfusion.

Both pre- and post-capillary sphincters are constricted by sympathetic stimulation so that flow through the capillary bed ceases. Eventually, local hypoxia and the accumulation of acid metabolites cause relaxation of the precapillary sphincters while the post-capillary sphincters remain constricted. In this way blood accumulates and stagnates in the capillaries. Vascular damage, extravasation and intravascular coagulation occur and may eventually result in irreversible tissue destruction.

It is the object of therapy to interrupt this sequence before irreversible damage has occurred.

REFERENCES

BRADLEY R.D. (1977) *Studies in Acute Heart Failure.* Edward Arnold, London.
BRADLEY R.D., JENKINS B.S., & BRANTHWAITE M.A. (1971) Myocardial function in acute glomerulonephritis. *Cardiovascular Research* **5**, 223.
BRAUNWALD E. (1965) The control of ventricular function in man. *Br. Heart J.* **27**, I.
JENKINS B.S., BRANTHWAITE M.A. & BRADLEY R.D. (1973) Cardiac function following open heart surgery: the relation between the performance of the two sides of the heart. *Cardiovascular Research* **7**, 297.
ROSS J. JR. & BRAUNWALD E. (1964) Studies on Starling's law of the heart. IX: the effects of impending venous return on performance of the normal and failing human left ventricle. *Circulation* **30**, 719.
SARNOFF S.J. & BERGLUND E. (1954) Ventricular function. I. Starling's law of the heart studied by means of right and left ventricular function curves in the dog. *Circulation* **9**, 706.
SHABETAI R., FOWLER N.D. & GUNTHEROTH W.G. (1970) The hemodynamics of cardiac tamponade and constrictive pericarditis. *Amer. J. Cardiol* **26**, 480.
STARLING E.H. (1918) *The Linrace Lecture on the Law of the Heart. Given at Cambridge.* Longman & Green, London.

CHAPTER 5

Low Cardiac Output

After cardiac surgery a low cardiac output may be due to many causes or combinations of causes. The blood volume may be too low. Accumulation of fluid in the pericardium may cause tamponade. Cardiac failure may occur from myocardial damage caused before or during surgery or be precipitated by dysrhythmias, acidosis, electrolyte imbalance or hypoxia. A low cardiac output occurring late in the postoperative period may be due to pulmonary embolism.

The clinical appearances of a low cardiac output are the result of inadequate perfusion of the tissues and vasoconstriction and are common to all these complications, but each cause has in addition its own characteristic physical signs. An accurate diagnosis is essential because the therapeutic measures necessary for one complication may be contraindicated for another.

In this chapter the clinical diagnosis of a low output is considered first, followed by the differential diagnosis of its causes. Treatment of a low cardiac output and its individual causes is discussed separately, and a summary of management is included at the end.

1. Clinical Diagnosis of a Low Cardiac Output

Under stress of a low cardiac output, the body attempts to preserve an adequate central blood pressure for perfusion of vital organs by reflex vasoconstriction in the skin, mucosa and abdominal viscera.

The diagnosis of a low cardiac output depends on recognition of poor perfusion of individual tissues, such as the skin, kidneys and brain. The blood flows more slowly than normally through the tissues which extract more oxygen so that its venous saturation falls. The tissues become hypoxic, anaerobic metabolism begins and acid metabolites accumulate in the blood.

a. GENERAL APPEARANCE

Restlessness and anxiety occur as the cerebral blood flow falls. The face becomes pale with a tinge of peripheral cyanosis of the nose, cheeks and ears. The skin is cold and later often sweaty.

49

b. FEET AND HANDS

Vasoconstriction gives rise to a pale, cool skin with constricted veins on the dorsum of the feet, absent dorsalis pedis and posterior tibial pulses and progressive peripheral cyanosis of feet and knees. A useful index of the progress of the cardiac output is the level of the 'temperature gradient', a term used to describe the level in the legs at which the skin changes from being warm to being cold. If the toe temperature is being monitored, the difference between it and the central 'core' temperature either fails to narrow after the patient's return from surgery or will start to widen. The core temperature rises as vasoconstriction prevents heat loss through the skin; the toe temperature falls from reduced skin perfusion. As the cardiac output improves, the temperature gradient moves towards the toes and finally disappears. The feet become warm and pink, the veins on the dorsum dilate and fill, and the arterial pulses become easily palpable again.

Vasoconstriction as a sign of low cardiac output is not reliable immediately after the patient's return from the operating theatre when it may be due to hypothermia, pain or anxiety. Severe tricuspid regurgitation also invalidates this sign because cutaneous vasodilatation may occur in spite of a low cardiac output.

c. RESPIRATORY AND PULSE RATES

If the patient is not on an artificial ventilator, the respiratory rate increases. If the patient is being ventilated, he may begin to 'fight' the ventilator. The heart rate also tends to increase. All beats may not reach the periphery, which makes the radial pulse unreliable in the presence of a low cardiac output.

d. BLOOD PRESSURE

The systolic blood pressure is not a reliable index of cardiac output but hypotension in the presence of vasoconstriction is of serious significance as it means that all measures taken by the body to sustain the blood pressure are failing.

Intra-arterial blood pressure measurement is more reliable than a sphygmomanometer cuff in the presence of severe vasoconstriction because the pulse pressure, the area under the pressure pulse and the rate of rise of pressure are better indices of the cardiac output than the systolic pressure. The critical level of systolic blood pressure is about 80 mmHg unless vasodilating drugs have been given.

e. VENOUS PRESSURE

The right atrial (or central venous) and left atrial (or wedge) pressures may be high or low depending on the cause of the low cardiac output. They are therefore of no value in diagnosing the low cardiac output itself.

f. URINE OUTPUT

The best single sign of a low cardiac output is reduction of urine output below the acceptable minimum of $\frac{1}{2}$ ml/kg/hr (30 ml/hr in an adult) because of the reduced renal perfusion. A low recorded urine volume may be due to a blocked urinary catheter, which should be changed if there is any doubt about its patency. Another cause is acute tubular necrosis of the kidneys, a diagnosis that is difficult to make in the presence of a low cardiac output but which is suggested by red cells and casts in the urine and continuing oliguria when the cardiac output increases.

g. BLOOD GAS ANALYSIS

The *partial pressure of oxygen* in the arterial blood (Pa_{O_2}) tends to drop as the cardiac output falls because the venous return to the lungs becomes more desaturated and some flows through the capillaries of collapsed alveoli to mix with oxygenated blood returning from the lungs. Such a drop is usual after cardiac surgery and is progressive until approximately the third day when the P_{O_2} begins to rise again. The fall is accentuated by a low cardiac output (Fig. 5.1). Hypoxia increases the pulmonary vascular resistence, which may already be high, and so cause right heart failure and decrease the cardiac output further.

A mixed venous sample of blood from, ideally, the pulmonary artery or, if this is not possible, the right atrium will show a reduction in oxygen saturation and tension. Comparison with the Pa_{O_2} allows the widened arteriovenous oxygen difference to be estimated as more oxygen is extracted by the tissues from the blood flowing sluggishly through them. A venous sample taken from a catheter with its tip in the IVC is unreliable because of the effects of streaming, as well oxygenated blood from the kidneys mixes poorly with desaturated blood from the limbs and minor alterations in the position of the catheter tip make for considerable changes in oxygen saturation.

The *partial pressure of carbon dioxide* (P_{CO_2}) may also fall, because rapid, shallow breathing tends to accompany a low cardiac output in a patient breathing spontaneously. The importance of this observation is that a normal or low P_{CO_2} does not preclude the use of positive pressure ventilation because the increase in available oxygen from the hyperventilation is less than the oxygen used in the increased work of the respiratory muscles. Positive pressure ventilation may then be indicated in spite of the low P_{CO_2} to spare the heart the extra work of hyperventilation.

The *standard bicarbonate and pH* of the blood fall as anaerobic metabolism

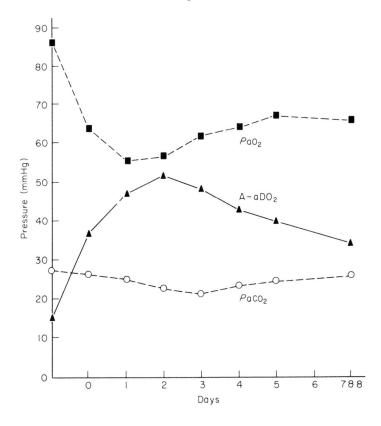

Fig. 5.1. Graph of blood gas analysis for the first week after aortic valve surgery. The partial pressure of oxygen (Pao_2) falls and the gradient between alveolar and arterial oxygen tension (A-aDO$_2$) rises showing the increased shunting of venous blood through underventilated alveoli. This change begins to correct itself by the third postoperative day. Note that the partial pressure of CO$_2$ ($Paco_2$) remains consistently below normal throughout (reprinted by permission from Fordham (1965) Thorax)

in the poorly perfused tissues causes acid metabolites to accumulate in the blood. Metabolic acidosis decreases the effectiveness of catecholamines and reduces myocardial contractility. The pulmonary vascular resistance also rises with a fall in pH which may reduce the cardiac output further.

h. MEASUREMENT OF CARDIAC OUTPUT

Direct measurement of the cardiac output is particularly valuable in the diagnosis and management of a low cardiac output. Many methods of assessment have been evaluated—dye dilution, extractable electromagnetic flow probes, Fick principle—but in the immediate postoperative period the thermodilution method of cardiac output estimation is the most practical and has been widely adopted throughout the world. The equipment is simple, reliable and commercially available and the output studies are rapidly repeatable. In this technique a cold bolus of saline is injected into the vena cava or right atrium, mixes with the venous return and the drop in temperature is recorded in the pulmonary artery by a small thermistor or a Swann–Ganz or other catheter floated into it before or after surgery. From the magnitude and shape of the temperature curve recorded, a small computer in the equipment calculates the cardiac output. This is repeated three times and the mean output estimated.

A cardiac output in a 70 kg man (1.73 m^2) below 1 l/min requires urgent correction within ten minutes if death is not to ensue: below 1.5 l/min has to be corrected within days: a flow above 2 l/min is adequate. A stroke work, calculated by multiplying the cardiac output by the 'developed pressure' in the ventricle, the mean aortic pressure minus the mean left atrial pressure, below 13 g/m (stroke work index 7.5 g/m/m) indicates a rapidly deteriorating situation if not quickly improved.

2. Differential Diagnosis of the Causes of a Low Cardiac Output

The important differentiating features in the diagnosis of the cause of a low cardiac output include the level and wave form of the right and left atrial venous pressures, the character of the arterial pulse, the ECG, the chest radiograph and the packed cell volume. Low atrial pressures suggest hypovolaemia or vasodilatation as the cause of the low output. High atrial pressures suggest tamponade (both atria), cardiac failure (either atrium) or pulmonary embolism (right atrium). In practice, hypovolaemia and tamponade are looked for first and dysrhythmias identified from the electrocardiogram, after which cardiac failure becomes the most likely cause of a persistently low cardiac output. Pulmonary embolism is considered when the major causes of a low cardiac output have been excluded. Adrenal failure is so rare a cause of a low cardiac output that it barely deserves consideration.

a. LOW BLOOD VOLUME (hypovolaemia)

A low central venous pressure may be due to loss of blood, plasma or water from the vascular tree, or to vasodilatation making the blood volume inadequate for the increased size of the vascular bed. The haemodynamic abnormalities associated with hypovolaemia are considered on page 43.

(i) AETIOLOGY OF A LOW CENTRAL VENOUS PRESSURE

1. *Haemorrhage*
Haemorrhage uncorrected by blood replacement is the usual cause of a low central venous pressure in the postoperative period. Inadequate haemostasis

is the most common cause of haemorrhage, mainly because the definition of 'inadequate' varies with the type of surgery being performed. Short operations, such as a mitral valvotomy or closure of an atrial septal defect leaving the patient with a low venous pressure, need relatively little attention to haemostasis. Long operations, such as multiple valve replacement after a previous mitral valvotomy or resection of a dissecting aneurysm of the aorta using profound hypothermia, require meticulous attention to haemostasis.

Decreased coagulability of the blood is the other main factor in postoperative haemorrhage. Its aetiology is considered fully in Chapter 13.

2. *Loss of water*

Large volumes of Ringer's lactate (Hartmann's solution) are commonly used for haemodilution during extracorporeal circulation in order to save blood. Water enters the extracellular space, which includes the vascular space, and is usually passed by the kidneys early in the postoperative period. If large volumes of urine are passed rapidly, the loss of water will reduce the blood volume.

Later in the postoperative period, dehydration may occur due to the overenthusiastic use of diuretics. The fluid balance chart over the preceding days shows a progressive negative fluid balance with output exceeding input. The tongue may be dry and the skin inelastic. The packed cell volume (haematocrit) rises progressively as a consequence of the haemoconcentration. Reduction in urine output is not a good index of dehydration after cardiac surgery because the reduced extracellular fluid volume is itself usually caused by excessive use of diuretics. If the patient can be weighed, a marked weight loss will be recorded compared with the preoperative weight.

Venous pressure catheters have often been removed by the time such fluid volume depletion occurs. If it is suspected, insertion of a central venous catheter will reveal a low or negative central venous pressure which responds to giving fluid.

3. *Vasodilatation*

A blood volume that may have been adequate for a given degree of venous tone may become inadequate if vasodilatation occurs, due to the increase in size of the venous capacitance vessels. Such vasodilatation may require substantially greater volume replacement in order that satisfactory filling pressures for the ventricles may be maintained.

The causes of vasodilatation after cardiac surgery are not always clear. Vasoconstriction is common in the period immediately after return of the patient to the intensive care unit due to several causes which include a low cardiac output, hypothermia, pain and anxiety. Vasodilatation occurs as the cardiac output rises. The patient becomes warmer and sedation while relieving pain and anxiety also relaxes venous tone. If vasodilator drugs, e.g. sodium nitroprusside, are being given to diminish the afterload of the ventricle or reduce hypertension, the central venous pressure may fall markedly.

(ii) DIAGNOSIS OF A LOW EFFECTIVE BLOOD VOLUME

1. *Clinical appearance*

A low blood volume causes vasoconstriction with low venous pressures unless the cause of the low effective blood volume is diminution of venous tone. There are therefore two clinical pictures. In one the patient is vasoconstricted, peripherally cyanosed, often with only a slightly reduced arterial pressure (Fig. 5.2), while in the other the patient is pink and warm but with marked hypotension. The venous pressures, both central and left atrial, are low and may be below zero when measured from the sternal angle.

HYPOVOLAEMIA / CONCEALED HAEMORRHAGE

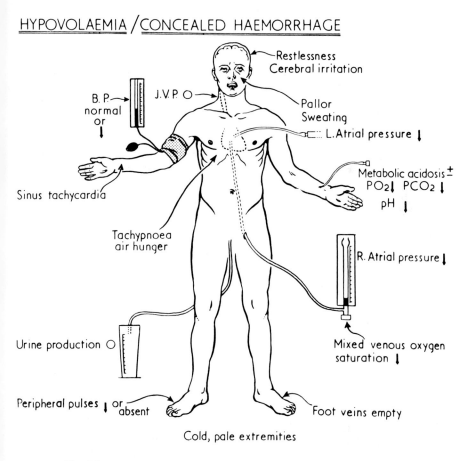

Fig. 5.2. Low blood volume. Diagram of the clinical picture (see text).

2. *Blood balance chart*

Measurement of blood loss and replacement on the blood balance chart may show blood replacement to have been less than or little more than the blood loss, unless haemorrhage has occurred into the pleura, mediastinum, abdomen or retroperitoneal tissues and has not been recognised. This is suggested when the blood balance chart shows a large positive balance with the atrial pressures still low.

3. *Evidence of haemorrhage from chest drains or on the chest radiograph*

There may be continuous or intermittent haemorrhage from chest drains and the chest radiograph may show an accumulation of blood in the pleural cavity or mediastinum.

Haemorrhage occurring in the presence of a normal clotting mechanism is suggested by drains becoming intermittently blocked with clot, a dry wound and venepuncture sites, and normal tests of the coagulation mechanism. Haemorrhage is sometimes due to abnormal clotting factors in the blood, the most common derangements being inadequate reversal of heparin or increased fibrinolysins. Absent or minimal clotting in chest drains, wounds oozing blood, prolonged bleeding after arterial and venepunctures, and abnormal haematological tests suggest that the haemorrhage is associated with clotting abnormalities which are considered fully in Chapter 13. Haematological tests may be normal, however, even though there is frank clinical evidence of lack of effective clotting.

4. *Rapid transfusion test*

Rapid transfusion of a small quantity of blood (50 ml in a child, 200 ml in an adult) produces a sharp, though temporary, improvement in blood pressure and urine volume if the cause of the low cardiac output is a low blood volume.

b. TAMPONADE

Tamponade is more common and more dangerous after cardiac surgery than is usually appreciated. Slight or intermittent drainage from pericardial or anterior mediastinal drains does not exclude bleeding, because the tubes may be blocked by blood clot. The classical physical signs of tamponade are seldom present in their entirety and may be considerably varied by loculated collections of clot. Even at postmortem, death due to tamponade often passes unrecognised because small collections of blood in the pericardium are ignored when the heart is collapsed, whereas they may have been critical during life.

(i) AETIOLOGY OF TAMPONADE

Tamponade is due to compression of the heart by fluid or clot in the pericardium or anterior mediastinum. The haemodynamic abnormalities are considered on page 44.

Acute tamponade after cardiac surgery is usually due to haemorrhage combined with inadequate pericardial drainage. Bleeding into a closed pericardium need not be considerable to produce a critical alteration in the clinical state, particularly if the heart is dilated from cardiac failure or overtransfusion. Tamponade due to bleeding into the pericardium usually occurs within 48 hours of operation but may sometimes happen days or even weeks later if anticoagulants have been given. The diagnosis has therefore to be borne particularly in mind if a fit patient deteriorates late in the postoperative period.

Chronic tamponade may occur in the post-pericardiotomy syndrome, due to serous fluid collection in the pericardium weeks or even months after operation.

(ii) DIAGNOSIS OF TAMPONADE (Fig. 5.3)

TAMPONADE

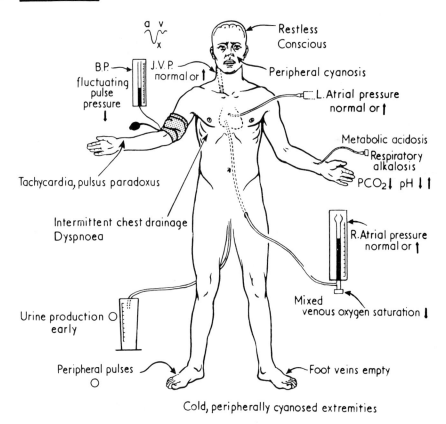

Fig. 5.3. Tamponade. Diagram of the clinical picture (see text).

The clinical picture of acute tamponade is of a fluctuating but gradually downhill course as the degree of tamponade varies from time to time as blood and serum leak from the pericardium or anterior mediastinum into the pleura or chest drains. The diagnosis of the chronic tamponade of the postpericardiotomy syndrome is considered on page 196.

1. *Raised venous pressure with systolic descent*
Both right and left atrial pressures are raised, with the dominant venous pulse wave being a systolic descent as blood ejected from the ventricle makes room for venous blood to enter the rigid pericardial compartment (Fig. 5.3).

2. *Fluctuating but generally falling blood pressure*
The blood pressure fluctuates, improving and deteriorating spasmodically, but the general tendency is downwards with a diminishing pulse pressure.

3. *Pulsus paradoxus*
The pulse has a small pulse pressure and volume with marked pulsus paradoxus, the pulse disappearing virtually completely during inspiration. A lesser degree of paradox with a drop of systolic pressure of up to 15 mmHg on inspiration is normal after any form of cardiac surgery and is not diagnostic of tamponade. The pattern of pulsus paradoxus is reversed by positive pressure ventilation, when the pulse disappears during expiration and improves on inspiration. Large intrapleural pressure swings, as in asthma, also produce a pulsus paradoxus.

4. *Echocardiography*
The presence of fluid between the ventricular cavities and the pericardium or sternum can be demonstrated by echocardiography. Smaller amounts of clot which may be clinically significant, may not be easily identified however, particularly if located laterally.

5. *Radio-opaque dye or CO_2 injection into the right atrium*
If angiographic equipment is available in the ITU, injection of radio-opaque dye into the right atrium will show a separation of the atrial cavity from the pericardial silhouette. With the patient in the lateral position, right side uppermost, injection of 25 ml of CO_2 will similarly reveal this separation.

6. *A conscious, pulseless patient*
A belated diagnosis of tamponade can sometimes be made when the patient becomes pulseless but remains conscious, the lack of pulsation in the carotid artery being due to the low pulse pressure.

(c) CARDIAC FAILURE

The incidence of low cardiac output due to cardiac failure has been markedly

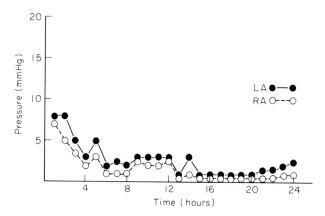

Fig. 5.4. Chart of left and right atrial pressures during the first 24 postoperative hours showing a 'normal' relationship between the two. These patients tend to have good myocardial contractility but occasionally this relationship occurs when both ventricles are equally poor. The atrial pressures are measured in mmHg from the sternal angle.

reduced by better myocardial preservation, particularly with cold cardio-plegia, in recent years.

Good myocardial contractility after cardiac surgery is shown by the heart's ability to maintain an adequate cardiac output with low filling pressures and with the mean left atrial pressure keeping its normal relationship some 3 mmHg above the right (Fig. 5.4). Cardiac failure can be defined as a state in which the heart fails to maintain an adequate circulation for the needs of the body despite a sufficient ventricular filling pressure and an adequate rate (Chapter 4). The ventricular function curve of the failing ventricle is flatter than normal (Fig. 4.3) so that the same stroke volume as the other ventricle is achieved but at a higher filling pressure.

The two ventricles may fail separately, although left ventricular failure will eventually compromise the right ventricle also. The diagnosis of cardiac failure may have to be made by exclusion—if there are no signs of haemorrhage, tamponade, dysrhythmias or pulmonary embolism, the assumption is that cardiac failure is the cause of the low output.

(i) DIAGNOSIS OF CARDIAC FAILURE
Failure of each ventricle is considered separately although both may fail together.

1. *Left ventricular failure* (Figs. 5.5–7)
A lesion that may be associated with left ventricular failure—aortic or mitral valve disease, systemic hypertension, myocardial damage or ischaemia—will usually be present (Figs. 5.5–5.7).

(a) *Raised left atrial pressure.* The left atrial pressure is high, with a dominant 'y' descent, and the right atrial pressure is well below the left (Figs. 5.8–5.9). The left atrial pressure may be consistently higher than the right but sometimes the relationship between them may fluctuate. A large 'v' wave of functional mitral incompetence may be seen on the left atrial pressure trace. The left ventricular function curve will have a flatter slope than normal with a smaller rise in stroke volume and work in relation to increases of atrial pressure (Fig. 4.3).

(b) *Pulsus alternans.* Pulsus alternans, an alternate larger and smaller pulse, may appear.

CARDIAC FAILURE – LEFT VENTRICULAR

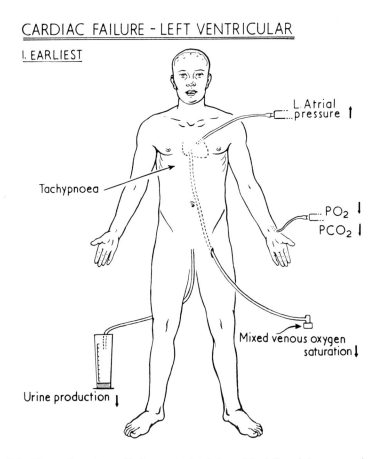

Fig. 5.5. The earliest signs of left ventricular failure. The left atrial pressure rises, and hyperventilation keeps the PCO_2 at or below normal. The PO_2 falls due to increased shunting of more desaturated venous blood through underventilated alveoli. Urine output usualy falls though occasionally there may be increased urinary production in the early stages. Toe temperature falls.

(c) *Tacky sputum, stiff lungs and pulmonary venous congestion on chest x-ray.*
The sputum is tacky and the lungs stiff. The respiratory rate is fast and the
alae nasi move if the patient is breathing spontaneously. Cheyne–Stokes
respiration may occur. The inflation pressure is high if he is being ventilated
artificially. The Po_2 falls.

A chest radiograph shows venous congestion and enlarged pulmonary
veins around the hilum. Raising the left atrial pressure too high by blood
transfusion on the assumption that the ventricular function curve is steep is
not uncommon if the right atrial pressure alone is monitored in the immediate
postoperative period and the possibility of a disparity between the two atrial
pressures ignored. The typical clinical picture of pulmonary oedema then
appears with crepitations in the lungs and the 'bat's wing' of frank pulmonary
oedema spreading from the hilum on the chest x-ray.

CARDIAC FAILURE - LEFT VENTRICULAR
2. EARLY

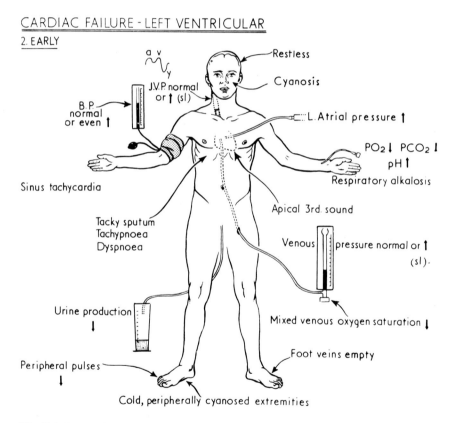

Fig. 5.6. Later signs of left ventricular failure. The patient becomes restless and
peripherally cyanosed, the feet become cold and vasoconstricted. The right atrial
pressure rises slightly and a third sound may become audible at the apex. Metabolic
acidosis tends to appear.

(d) *Auscultation of heart.* There may be a third sound at the apex which is loudest on expiration, though this is often obscured by pericardial noise in the first few postoperative days. The heart sounds are softer than normal. If a prosthetic mitral valve has been inserted, the interval between the aortic second sound and the opening sound will be short as the raised left atrial pressure reduces the time that the left ventricular pressure takes to fall to atrial level (reduced isovolumic relaxation period).

2. *Right ventricular failure* (Fig. 5.10)

A lesion that may be associated with right ventricular failure—a right ventriculotomy, pulmonary stenosis, pulmonary hypertension, pulmonary embolism or severe tricuspid regurgitation—is usually present.

(a) *Raised right atrial (central venous) pressure.* The central venous pressure is high, the left atrial pressure lower (Fig. 5.11). A large 'v' wave of functional

CARDIAC FAILURE - LEFT VENTRICULAR

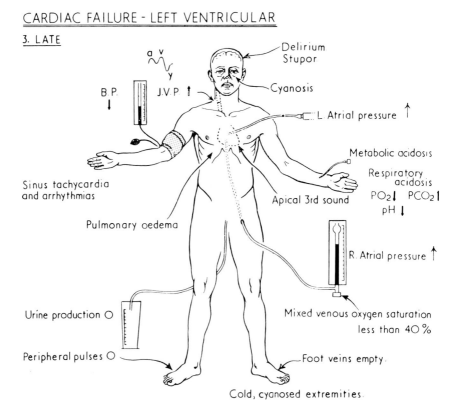

3. LATE

- a v y
- B.P. ↓
- J.V.P. ↑
- Delirium Stupor
- Cyanosis
- L. Atrial pressure ↑
- Metabolic acidosis
- Respiratory acidosis
- Sinus tachycardia and arrhythmias
- Apical 3rd sound
- PO_2↓ PCO_2↑ pH ↓
- Pulmonary oedema
- R. Atrial pressure ↑
- Urine production O
- Mixed venous oxygen saturation less than 40 %
- Peripheral pulses O
- Foot veins empty.
- Cold, cyanosed extremities.

Fig. 5.7. Classical left ventricular failure with signs of a very low cardiac output and pulmonary oedema is a late clinical picture. If treatment is delayed until this stage is evident, the situation is often irreversible.

tricuspid regurgitation may be seen on the central venous trace and in the neck. A pulsatile liver may be felt.

(b) *Rising haematocrit.* The packed cell volume gradually rises as fluid transudes into the tissue spaces because of the high systemic venous pressure. The PCV may reach 50–60%, which will increase viscosity and slow flow in the micro-circulation.

(c) *Auscultation of the heart.* A third sound which is loudest on inspiration may be audible at the left sternal edge. If the operation has been a pulmonary valvotomy or infundibular resection (Brock operation), right ventricular failure may be due to increased tone of the infundibulum which tends to follow anxiety or pain. The pulmonary systolic ejection murmur then becomes shorter, and may disappear altogether in extreme cases.

(d) *Dependent oedema and ascites.* Sacral oedema appears after a lag of a day or more. Oedema only appears when excess extracellular fluid exceeds 3 l and is therefore a late sign of failure. Shifting dullness in the abdomen suggests ascites though this is also a late sign. Weight gain is a better index of fluid retention but weighing the patient is impractical early after operation (Fig. 5.17).

3. *Failure of both ventricles*
Not uncommonly, the myocardial contractility of both ventricles is reduced equally and the clinical appearances of both right and left ventricular failure are seen. The flat and almost superimposed ventricular function curves under these circumstances mean that right and left atrial mean pressures are similar. Poor right ventricular function, however, makes pulmonary oedema less likely.

d. DYSRHYTHMIAS

Any rhythm other than sinus rhythm is termed a dysrhythmia. Sinus bradycardia or tachycardia has also to be considered in this context. When atrial systole occurs just before ventricular contraction (0.12–0.18 seconds before), the ventricle is optimally filled so that it generates its optimal force of contraction. Any other rhythm prevents this and tends to reduce the stroke volume, which may be critical in cardiac patients.

Dysrhythmias are due either to an ectopic pacemaker that overrides the sino-atrial node or to poor or blocked conduction of the impulse through the atrio-ventricular node, bundle of His or Purkinje system. If the abnormal impulse arises in or above the A-V node, the dysrhythmia is termed supraventricular and this term may be taken to include atrial flutter, atrial fibrillation, nodal rhythm and other dysrhythmias. The QRS complex is usually the same as that of preceding sinus beats. Ventricular dysrhythmias are caused by an irritable focus in the ventricles. The QRS complex is then always abnormal because the ventricular fibres are depolarised in an abnormal order. Either type of dysrhythmia may be associated with too slow or too fast a ventricular rate.

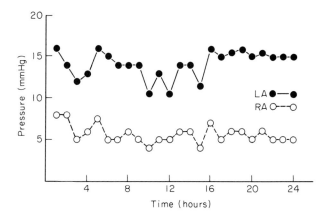

Fig. 5.8. Chart of left and right atrial pressures in a patient with poor left ventricular function. The left atrial pressure is consistently higher than the right.

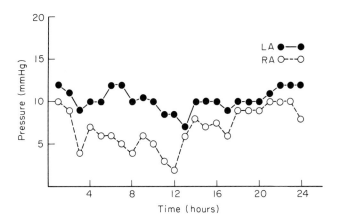

Fig. 5.9. Chart of left and right atrial pressures in a patient with poor left ventricular function but in whom the relationship between the atrial pressures fluctuated widely. This pattern is common after valve replacement surgery.

Heart block occurs when the depolarising impulse is not conducted from the SA node to the ventricle. First degree heart block occurs when the passage of the depolarising impulse is slower than normal (long P-R interval): in second-degree block there is failure of the ventricles to follow each atrial contraction, and in complete heart block the atria and ventricles beat entirely independently with a slow ventricular rate (atrio-ventricular dissociation) (p. 66).

CARDIAC FAILURE – RIGHT VENTRICULAR

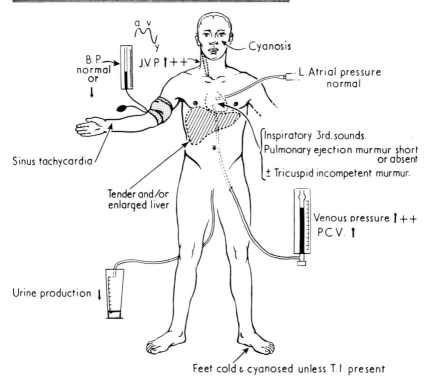

Fig. 5.10. Right ventricular failure. The clinical picture is of congestive failure with or without the signs of tricuspid incompetence.

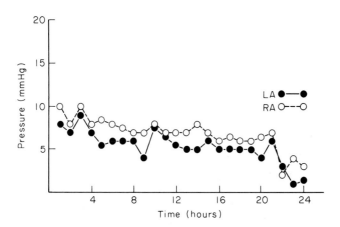

Fig. 5.11. Chart of left and right atrial pressures in a patient with poor right ventricular contractility. The right atrial pressure is consistently higher than the left.

(i) AETIOLOGY OF DYSRHYTHMIAS

1. *Supraventricular dysrhythmias*

The cause of supraventricular dysrhythmias is seldom obvious but they may be precipitated by a period of low cardiac output, metabolic acidosis, poor myocardial contractility, hypoxia, pericardial involvement, pulmonary collapse, pulmonary emboli and heart failure. Damage to the sino-atrial node by the insertion of atrial cannulae too close to it or injury to the branches of the right coronary artery to the SA and A-V node may be associated with postoperative supraventricular dysrhythmias. Overdistension of the atria is a significant cause.

The aetiology of paroxysmal atrial tachycardia with variable block, where there is rapid atrial activity with only slightly abnormal P waves and a 3 or 4:1 blocked ventricular response is often due to over-digitalization and may be precipitated by a low plasma potassium content. Any atrial dysrhythmia can be produced by digoxin—nodal bradycardia may precede tachycardia for instance.

2. *Ventricular dysrhythmias*

After cardiac surgery ventricular dysrhythmias are due to an ectopic focus in an irritable myocardium. The myocardium may have been damaged by poor myocardial preservation at the time of surgery, by coronary artery trauma, thrombosis of grafts or embolism, by previous myocardial infarction or by low coronary flow due to a low cardiac output. Its irritability is also increased by hypoxia and by digitalis, particularly if the serum potassium is low which is a common cause of dysrhythmias even if no digitalis has been given. The fall in the incidence of troublesome ventricular dysrhythmias has been one of the features of cold cardioplegic myocardial preservation.

3. *Heart block*

Heart block occurring after cardiac surgery is commonly due to damage to the conducting fibres at surgery. Operations placing the bundle of His particularly at risk are closure of ventricular or ostium primum atrial septal defects, aortic valve replacement of heavily calcified valves, or tricuspid valve replacement. Operations on corrected transposition of the great arteries are hazardous in this respect. Heart block may, however, occur spontaneously without surgical damage to the conducting fibres if there is underlying fibrosis or coronary artery disease. Latent heart block may be unmasked by uraemia, digitalis intoxication, lignocaine, quinidine or severe myocardial failure, and temporary heart block has become more common since the introduction of cold cardioplegia for myocardial preservation at surgery.

(ii) DIAGNOSIS OF DYSRHYTHMIAS

Dysrhythmias are diagnosed from the electrocardiogram. The wave form of the venous pulse may also be useful at times. All patients with a low cardiac output are constantly monitored with an ECG oscilloscope because, even when dysrhythmias are not the cause of the low output, they often develop if coronary perfusion and oxygenation fall and metabolic acidosis appears.

Diagnosis of the specific dysrhythmia is made from the ECG by assessment of the relation of the P wave to the QRS complex, the shape of the QRS complex, and the presence of tachycardia, bradycardia, ectopic beats or complete irregularity of the pulse. Some of the more common dysrhythmias encountered after cardiac surgery are considered below.

1. *Absent or abnormal P waves*

In nodal rhythm the atria and ventricles beat together and the P wave is buried in the QRS complex (Fig. 5.12). In addition 'cannon' waves, marked systolic waves, may be seen on the venous dynamic pressure trace. These waves raise the mean venous pressure. In atrial fibrillation no P waves are seen, the base line is wavy and the QRS complex occurs irregularly (Fig.

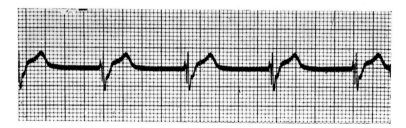

Fig. 5.12. Nodal rhythm.

5.13). There will be no 'a' wave on the venous pressure traces. In atrial flutter, sawtoothed flutter waves are present at a rate of about 300 per minute and there is usually a degree of A-V block (e.g. 4:1 block means one QRS complex to 4 flutter waves (Fig. 5.14). In paroxysmal atrial tachycardia with varying block, the atrial rate is between 160 and 220 but the waves look normal and the degree of block tends to vary.

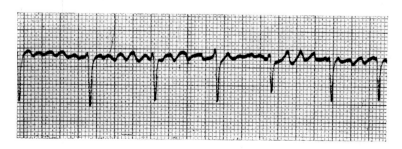

Fig. 5.13. Atrial fibrillation.

2. *Broad QRS complex*

In right or left bundle branch block there is abnormal conduction in one or other bundle branch which causes delay in activation of part of the ventricle and broadens the QRS complex. In ventricular extrasystoles and tachycardia the origin of the impulse is in the ventricle rather than A-V node and this produces an abnormally broad QRS complex. Ventricular fibrillation causes totally variable waves. Gross potassium excess also causes widening of the QRS complex.

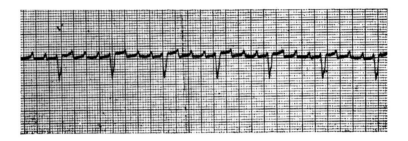

Fig. 5.14. Atrial flutter.

3. *Regular tachycardia*

In sinus tachycardia the P waves are usually visible but may sometimes be masked by the preceding T wave. In nodal tachycardia the P waves may notch the QRS. In ventricular tachycardia the QRS complex is wide. It is difficult to distinguish it from supraventricular tachycardia with left bundle branch block without special leads.

4. *Regular bradycardia*

In sinus bradycardia the P waves are normal and in nodal bradycardia they are inverted. In complete heart block there are regular P waves but completely dissociated, though regular, QRS complexes (Fig. 5.15).

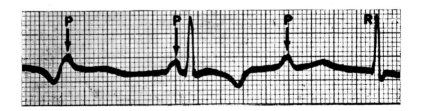

Fig. 5.15. Complete heart block.

5. *Ectopic beats*

When they arise in the atria (supraventricular), the QRS complex is usually normal for that patient. Nodal ectopic beats show inverted or absent P waves. The QRS complex is basically normal but may have a notch on it (Fig. 5.12). Ventricular ectopic beats show a wide QRS complex (Fig. 5.16). If an extrasystole occurs regularly after each normal beat, it is termed coupling or bigeminy and suggests a low serum potassium level. In the Wenckebach and reversed Wenckebach phenomenon the P-R interval progressively increases or decreases until a beat is dropped, when the cycle begins again.

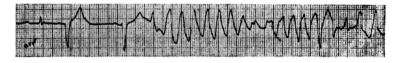

Fig. 5.16. Ventricular fibrillation preceded by two ventricular ectopic beats.

6. *Irregularity of the rate of the QRS complex*

In sinus arrhythmia there are normal P waves and QRS complexes but the heart rate slows on expiration. In atrial fibrillation the baseline is wavy but the QRS complexes are usually normal (Fig. 5.13). In ventricular fibrillation there is a wavy line with no obvious QRS complex (Fig. 5.16). In variable block, the QRS complex only follows some of the P waves.

e. PULMONARY EMBOLISM

Pulmonary embolism after cardiac surgery usually follows thrombosis in the veins of the legs or, rarely, the pelvis, but clot may also come from suture lines, prosthetic material or infarcts in the right side of the heart and ventricular septum.

In normal patients, only a massive pulmonary embolus occluding 60–80% of the pulmonary vascular tree will cause a persistently low cardiac output, but smaller emboli can precipitate failure after cardiac surgery. Massive pulmonary embolism is extremely rare in the immediate post-bypass period.

(i) DIAGNOSTIC FEATURES

1. *Sudden deterioration*

The patient's cardiac output deteriorates suddenly and he may complain of sudden severe dyspnoea and central chest pain.

2. *Right ventricular failure*

An acutely raised jugular venous or right atrial pressure, an increased right ventricular impulse and an inspiratory third heart sound at the left sternal edge are the signs of acute right ventricular overload.

3. *ECG*

The mean QRS axis shifts to the right compared with previous electrocardiograms and there is ST segment depression and T inversion. The $S_1Q_3T_3$ syndrome may occur—an S wave in lead I, Q wave in lead III with T inversion in the same lead—and cause confusion with inferior myocardial infarction.

4. *Pulmonary angiography and radioactive isotope scanning*

Injection of radio-opaque dye into the right heart outlining the pulmonary arteries is the only certain way of making the diagnosis and confirming its extent. The decision to do the investigation is difficult after major cardiac surgery on a seriously ill patient but has to be performed if there is real doubt about the diagnosis. Ventilation/perfusion lung scans with radioactive isotopes cause less circulatory disturbance but are less reliable if pulmonary complications such as atelectasis are also present.

f. ADRENAL EXHAUSTION

Adrenal exhaustion is a very rare cause of a low cardiac output but does occur after bilateral adrenal haemorrhage. It is also found in septicaemia. Accurate diagnosis is not possible but, if the possibility is considered, intravenous steroids may be given and can be lifesaving.

3. Treatment of a Low Cardiac Output

Once the cause of the low cardiac output has been diagnosed, therapy becomes relatively straightforward. The overall management of a patient with a low cardiac output is considered at the end of this section.

a. LOW BLOOD VOLUME

(i) TRANSFUSION OF BLOOD, PLASMA, WATER OR ELECTROLYTES

The treatment of a low blood volume is transfusion of the appropriate fluid—blood, plasma, plasma substitute or water and electrolytes depending on the haematocrit (packed cell volume). If the PCV is less than 45%, blood is transfused. If it is more than 45% and an estimate of the water balance excludes dehydration as the cause, plasma or a plasma substitute such as albumin in transfused. If dehydration is thought to be the cause of the raised PCV, 5% dextrose is given, with the addition of 0.18% saline if the sodium level is low.

Once the lower of the two venous pressures has reached 5–10 mmHg when measured from the sternal angle (15–20 mmHg from mid-chest level), a low blood volume can be excluded as the sole cause of the low cardiac output. A larger blood volume and a higher venous pressure may, however, be necessary in cardiac failure following surgery in order to raise the filling pressure of the failing ventricle and enable it to achieve an adequate stroke volume.

(ii) HAEMOSTASIS

If haemorrhage continues from chest drains, or blood accumulates in the pleura, pericardium or anterior mediastinum, a decision has first to be made as to whether it is occurring in the presence of a normal or abnormal clotting mechanism. If wounds and venepunctures are dry, clots are appearing in draining tubes and laboratory tests of coagulation are normal, haemorrhage is likely to be 'surgical' due to bleeding points neglected at the time of surgery.

The next decision is when to reopen the chest for haemostasis. Delay until large amounts of stored, citrated blood have been given and the blood volume has been allowed to fluctuate widely may result in the cardiac output being so low that cardiac, cerebral, renal or hepatic damage occurs before the bleeding is controlled and a consumptive coagulopathy may be initiated. If the patient bleeds more than 200 ml/hour for more than three hours, or bleeds 400 ml in any one hour, the chest is reopened for haemostasis.

Reopening a wound for haemorrhage can be dangerous. Induction of anaesthesia dilates the vascular system and the blood volume may then be inadequate. Reopening a lateral thoracotomy involves turning a patient on his side so that the weight of pleural or pericardial clot lays on the heart or compresses the lung. The plasma potassium level also may have risen to dangerous levels if suxamethonium is used for induction and if tissue perfusion has been poor and urine output reduced.

The patient is best transferred conscious onto the operating table with monitoring lines still connected to oscilloscopes. Better still, facilities should be available for operating under sterile conditions in the ITU. The patient is then not disturbed by movement, remains connected to the monitoring equipment and the operation is quicker. The surgeons scrub before anaesthesia is induced and the chest is opened as rapidly as possible afterwards and the clot evacuated and haemostasis achieved. Evacuation of all clot is an important part of the procedure because local fibrinolysins in clot promote bleeding. As soon as the main bleeding points are controlled, the cardiac output tends to improve markedly. Haemostasis has then to be meticulous because some degree of diminution of coagulation factors will have occurred during the transfusion of large quantities of stored blood.

(iii) CORRECTION OF ABNORMAL CLOTTING FACTORS

Evidence of an abnormal clotting mechanism—absence of clot in drainage tubes and bottles, oozing wounds and venepuncture sites, bruising, or abnormal clotting tests—demands correction of the abnormal clotting factor. If a specific abnormal factor is found, it is corrected as outlined in Chapter 13.

Usually, in spite of evidence of poor clotting, no specific coagulation abnormality can be found. Fresh frozen plasma and fresh blood are then the best general measures. Clotting factors, particularly platelets, diminish rapidly in effectiveness with time after drawing blood, and donors can be cross matched in advance of any operation particularly likely to be associated with haemorrhage, so that blood can be drawn and given immediately without the necessity for the 2 hour delay of cross matching. Platelet rich plasma is given if platelets are markedly diminished.

If blood is being given rapidly, calcium is given (2–5 ml of 20% calcium chloride, 0.5g $CaCl_2$) for each unit of ACD blood transfused if the patient is cold, has a low cardiac output or has hepatic damage, because the calcium which is necessary for coagulation may be fixed by the citrate content of the blood. At slower rates of transfusion of ACD blood, citrate is metabolized in the liver and calcium mobilised from bone so that coagulation is not affected. Calcium is nevertheless still best given in order to improve contractility.

b. TAMPONADE

Immediate evacuation of fluid and clotted blood from the pericardium is imperative once tamponade has been diagnosed.

(i) MILKING OF PERICARDIAL DRAINS
The chest drains are 'milked' continuously by the nurses with rollers or fingers while preparations are made to reopen the chest, because removing even a few ml of fluid may markedly improve the patient's condition.

(ii) REOPENING THE LOWER END OF A MEDIAN STERNOTOMY
Reopening the lower end of a median sternotomy wound and inserting two fingers and a sucker behind the sternum is occasionally life saving if the patient becomes moribund before arrangements have been completed for reopening the chest fully.

(iii) HAEMOSTASIS
The wound is reopened fully, clot evacuated and haemostasis achieved. Clot is removed from chest drains to allow them to drain freely again.

c. CARDIAC FAILURE

The management of cardiac failure involves paying attention to the three factors affecting the function of the ventricles—the preload, myocardial contractility and the afterload (Fig. 4.1)—and ensuring an adequate heart rate. In practice preload and heart rate are adjusted first, then myocardial contractility improved and finally afterload reduced.

(i) ENSURING AN OPTIMAL FILLING PRESSURE FOR THE VENTRICLES (PRELOAD)

Starling established in essence that the greater the filling pressure—in actuality the resting fibre length—the greater the force of contraction of the ventricle (page 39). The ventricle most under stress, left or right, will have the higher filling pressure initially. The mean atrial pressure of that side of the heart is raised slowly by transfusion of the appropriate fluid (page 70) until the stroke volume improves. The improvement is best measured directly with frequent cardiac output estimations but may be inferred by a rising urinary output and better skin perfusion. The mean atrial pressure (saline manometer or electrical measurement from a transducer) is unreliable in the presence of nodal rhythm, with its cannon waves, or mitral and tricuspid regurgitation with large 'v' waves. A dynamic trace to assess the end-diastolic pressure is invaluable in these instances. Otherwise, allowance has to be made for the raised mean pressures.

Cardiac output and pulmonary oedema are separate and contradictory problems during the management of postoperative cardiac failure. The highest acceptable right atrial (central venous) pressure is that which corresponds to a left atrial 'wedge' pressure of 20 mmHg measured from the sternal angle or 25–30 mmHg from mid-chest level. Even this maximum pressure must be reduced if the serum albumin level is low due to haemodilution after bypass or preoperative hepatic failure. A left atrial pressure of 12 mmHg will produce pulmonary oedema if the serum albumin is half normal.

If the left atrial (wedge) pressure is not being directly measured, tachypnoea, moving alae nasi, basal crepitations, a falling Po_2, increasing inflation pressure when on a ventilator or the appearance of a hilar flare on the chest x-ray will indicate an unacceptably high left ventricular filling pressure.

Attempts to raise cardiac output by raising the filling pressure become less and less effective as the function of the ventricle worsens. If the ventricular function curve is flat, a large rise of filling pressure will produce minimal or no improvement in stroke volume (Fig. 4.3).

((ii) MAINTAINING AN OPTIMAL HEART RATE

If the stroke volume is low, a faster than normal heart rate will help to maintain an adequate cardiac output. Increasing the rate however also increases the oxygen consumption of the heart and a balance has therefore to be drawn. A rate of 100/minute has been shown to be the optimum under these circumstances. An increased rate is achieved by the use of a chronotropic drug, such as isoprenaline, or a pacemaker.

1. *Isoprenaline (Isuprel)*

Isoprenaline may be given to maintain a heart rate of 90–100/min (page 41). The decision as to whether to use isoprenaline or a pacemaker to increase the heart rate depends mainly on individual units' preferences and experience, but in general isoprenaline is preferred if peripheral vasoconstriction is marked or if myocardial contractility requires to be enhanced, while the pacemaker is preferred if ventricular dysrhythmias are occurring.

2. *Pacemakers*

Pacemaker wires attached to atria or ventricles at the time of surgery, or inserted into the atrium or apex of the ventricle from an internal jugular, subclavian or axillary vein in the ITU, will keep the heart rate at any desired level. The ability to use a pacemaker is particularly valuable after cardiac surgery because digoxin can then be given liberally for its inotropic action without fear of producing an excessive bradycardia. Atrial pacemaking is used if the patient is in sinus rhythm because then the 'a' wave of atrial contraction has its proper relation to ventricular contraction (page 41). Ventricular pacemaking has to be used if A–V dissociation occurs unless equipment allowing sequential pacing of atria and ventricles is available, when it may be life saving.

(iii) IMPROVING MYOCARDIAL CONTRACTILITY

If raising the filling pressure to the highest acceptable level and maintaining the heart rate at 100 beats/minute fails to achieve an adequate cardiac output, the ventricular function curve is flatter because of poor myocardial contractility (Fig. 4.3). Inotropic drugs are then instituted to improve the contractility of the ventricles.

1. *Isoprenaline (Isuprel) and dopamine (Intropin)*

Isoprenaline improves myocardial contractility, raising the slope of the ventricular function curve so that the same filling pressure produces a larger stroke volume (page 40). It is best given by continuous intravenous infusion as in this way its effect can be regulated and rapidly changed when necessary.*

The isoprenaline is infused at a rate that achieves the desired effect, as

---

* A solution of 1 mg isoprenaline in 500 ml dextrose is infused, preferably into a central vein by an intravenous line that is separate from the fluid or blood transfusion lines. Use of a central vein precludes interruption of the infusion by thrombosis or kinking of limb veins and a separate line avoids excessive amounts of isoprenaline being flushed in by quantities of another fluid flowing in the same line. It can be given in a Buretrol paediatric microdrip set in which 4 microdrops = 1 normal drop, and 30 microdrops per minute ≡ 1 µg/min of isoprenaline ≡ 30 ml of fluid per hour. The microdrip set allows for fine adjustment of the infusion. If excessive volumes of fluid are being given by this dilution of isoprenaline, 1 mg is mixed in 100 ml in the Buretrol 100 ml bag (15 microdrops/min ≡ 2.5 µg isoprenaline/min ≡ 15 ml of fluid per hour). Even better control of isoprenaline infusion, with the use of smaller volumes of fluid, is achieved if a constant infusion pump is used.

judged by improvement of urine flow and skin perfusion or by direct measurement of the cardiac output. A tachycardia of more than 120/min or frequent ventricular dysrhythmias may occur and necessitate slowing the infusion rate. If isoprenaline fails to produce an effect, the cause may be metabolic acidosis which impairs the effects of catecholamines.

Dopamine* (Intropin) has a similar inotropic effect to isoprenaline but a less marked chronotropic effect. It is therefore valuable when the heart rate is already fast (e.g. atrial fibrillation or in children). It also specifically promotes a diuresis in its lower dose range which is valuable when urine output is low.

If any acidosis is corrected and isoprenaline or dopamine still fails to improve contractility, adrenaline (1 ml of 1:1000 in 500 ml dextrose) may be used in addition. A central venous line is then essential because extravasation of adrenaline may otherwise cause skin necrosis. Adrenaline increases the peripheral vascular resistance by inducing skin and abdominal visceral constriction and enables a small cardiac output to maintain an adequate central pressure for cerebral and renal perfusion. Its use is discontinued as soon as possible as the work of the heart is increased by the increased afterload: simultaneous use of sodium nitroprusside avoids this particular disadvantage.

If the rate of infusion of an inotropic drug is expressed as micrograms per minute (μg/min) rather than as drops/min, comparability of infusion of different strengths of solutions and different inotropes is facilitated. For comparable inotropic effect, approximately four times as much adrenaline is required as isoprenaline.

2. *Digoxin*

The important actions of digitalis glycosides (digoxin, digotoxin, lanatoside C, etc.) are improvement of myocardial contractility and delay of the passage of the impulse from atria to ventricles. The first effect is used in myocardial failure though it is minimal if isoprenaline or dopamine is also being given. The latter effect is particularly valuable when a rapid rate is being transmitted directly to the ventricles (e.g. atrial flutter and fibrillation).

Digoxin is probably the simplest drug to use because it is the most commonly used glycoside in Britain and experience with it is widespread.†

* 100 mg dopamine are made up to 100 ml with 5% dextrose in a Buretrol 100 ml giving set. 10 microdrops/min ≡ 1.65 μg/min. Better, in a 50 ml constant infusion pump, 200 mg dopamine are added to 45 ml 5% dextrose. 1 ml/hour ≡ 70 μg/min.

† The dose that will produce full digitalization in any individual patient cannot be predicted because individual sensitivity varies. The digitalizing dose of digoxin is approximately 0.9 mg/square metre of surface area or roughly 1.5 mg for the average adult with 0.25–0.5 mg as a daily maintenance dose. It is safer to give divided doses rather than a single large dose. Overdosage is then less likely because subsequent doses can be omitted if nausea or bradycardia appears. A regime of 0.5 mg 3 hourly for 3 doses, then 0.25 mg three times a day is safe for relatively rapid digitalization in an adult. Slower digitalization will be at about half this rate.

Digitoxin (Nativelle's digitalin) causes less nausea (0.1 mg is equivalent to 0.25 mg of digoxin) but its effects last longer and overdosage takes longer to correct.

Whatever the dosage rate chosen, further doses are discontinued if the toxic effects of digitalis appear—nausea, vomiting, bradycardia or ventricular dysrhythmias, etc. The plasma potassium level is checked because a low potassium potentiates the toxic effects of digitalis and may cause dangerous ventricular dysrhythmias.

Digoxin is safest when given orally, most dangerous when given intravenously. If oral administration is impossible, digoxin is best administered over 1 hour in an intravenous infusion. If toxic effects appear or the plasma potassium falls the infusion can be discontinued with the knowledge that no more will be absorbed. Intramuscular injections are poorly and unpredictably absorbed. As oral digoxin is only 60–80% absorbed, equivalent doses for parenteral routes should be reduced accordingly.

Renal failure with or without oliguria also calls for reduction of digoxin dosage because of reduced excretion of the drug. Raised blood urea and creatinine levels are indications for reduction in digoxin dosage because creatinine and digoxin clearance run parallel.

3. Calcium
Calcium may improve poor myocardial contractility dramatically but usually temporarily. Calcium is nevertheless valuable particularly if the plasma potassium level is high. 5 ml of 20% (0.5g) calcium chloride are given slowly intravenously, so as to avoid unpleasant vasodilatation, and repeated as necessary.

4. Other drugs
Glucose and insulin given intravenously force potassium into the cells and have been said to improve myocardial contractility. 50 u of insulin are added to 500 ml of 50% dextrose. 50 mmol of potassium chloride are added if the plasma potassium is normal or low. Ventricular dysrhythmias may be diminished though the effect on myocardial contractility is usually disappointing. This solution is given at a rate of 100 ml/hour or, in an emergency, as 100 ml rapidly. The left atrial pressure rises sharply, though temporarily, at the latter rate of infusion which may precipitate pulmonary oedema. The plasma level of potassium may fall dramatically in spite of the 50 mmol in the bottle and extra potassium is given if the plasma level falls below 4 mmol/l, which may cause a rebound to high levels when the glucose and insulin is discontinued. Serial potassium estimations are therefore essential when glucose and insulin are being infused, and are continued for 12 hours afterwards.

Glucagon has been shown to improve myocardial contractility and may be tried, but in our hands has not been markedly effective after cardiac surgery.

5. *Specific measures in failure of individual ventricles*

Left ventricular failure causes stiff lungs, tacky sputum and, finally, pulmonary oedema. Skilled physiotherapy may keep the bronchi clear but artificial ventilation with an endotracheal tube or tracheostomy is particularly valuable in left ventricular failure if it does not respond to simpler measures. The inflation pressure may rise to 50 cm H_2O or more but frank pulmonary oedema can usually be averted by positive pressure ventilation with a positive end-expiratory pressure.

Right ventricular failure causes a high systemic venous pressure with extravasation of fluid into the extracellular space and consequent haemoconcentration. Water can be kept in the vascular compartment and the PCV kept below 45% by transfusing double strength plasma or plasma substitute instead of blood to maintain the filling pressure of the right ventricle. Removing blood and replacing it with plasma with careful control of the atrial pressures is equally effective. Reducing tricuspid regurgitation by lowering the right atrial pressure sometimes improves the cardiac output and should be tried if there is evidence of gross tricuspid regurgitation. Blood is carefully removed from a venous line into a citrated transfusion container, so that it can be used again if necessary.

(iv) REDUCTION OF AFTERLOAD (VASODILATATION)

As soon as ventricular systole opens the aortic valve, the left ventricle is confronted with the peripheral resistance (impedance) of the aorta and arterioles (Fig. 4.1). The higher the impedance and aortic pressure, the greater is the work load on the ventricle. Vasodilator drugs can be used to reduce this afterload and so the oxygen consumption of the myocardium, while at the same time improving tissue perfusion by arteriolar dilatation.

Isoprenaline is a peripheral vasodilating drug, but, more specifically, sodium nitroprusside* or phentolamine (Rogitine)† may be given. Phentolamine is best used in boluses when the patient first returns from the operating theatre: nitroprusside by continuous infusion. The skin becomes pinker and warmer and the patient looks better with often an improved urinary flow. Aminophylline is occasionally useful also.

Vasodilator drugs are valuable in the patient who returns to the ITU tightly constricted, pale, peripherally cyanosed with a normal or higher than normal blood pressure. This clinical picture is seen not infrequently now that cold cardioplegia is allowing better myocardial preservation during surgery. Vasodilator drugs should be used with caution in the presence of a low cardiac output, as the stroke volume may be too small to maintain an adequate blood pressure in the face of the reduced impedance in spite of the

---

* Sodium nitroprusside is made up fresh in a solution of 50 mg (2 ml) added to 48 ml 5% dextrose and given at the rate of 50–150 μg/min to achieve the desired affect. Toxic overdosage is unlikely on this regime.

† Phentolamine (Rogitine) is given in boluses of 1 mg at a time.

tachycardia that usually accompanies their use. Coronary and renal blood flow may be reduced with sometimes fatal results.

A combination, however, of nitroprusside to lower the afterload, raising the preload (left and right atrial pressures), which will have fallen as the patient 'bleeds' into his own dilated vasculature, by transfusion, and adding an inotropic drug, e.g. dopamine or adrenaline, can be most effective in low cardiac output states, particularly when the left atrial pressure has been close to pulmonary oedema levels. This combination not infrequently proves life saving when all other measures have failed and has its greatest effect when the heart is large.

(v) REMOVAL OF EXCESS WATER AND SODIUM
Cardiac failure accentuates the usual postoperative sodium and water retention which may cause pulmonary and systemic oedema. Treatment is by restriction of sodium intake and promotion of a diuresis, taking care to replace potassium losses.

1. *Restriction of sodium and water intake*
The fluid replacement regime outlined in Chapter 9 (500 ml/m² on the first day, 800 ml/m² on the subsequent two days) is designed to prevent an excessive water or sodium load in the early postoperative period. Dextrose, rather than dextrose/saline, is used if any suggestion of cardiac failure is present. Water restriction is important early in the postoperative period, particularly when dilution perfusions have been used, because sodium retention always occurs, water is retained and the extracellular fluid volume is increased. Renal function may also be poor. Dextrose, rather than saline, is used to dilute drugs, and sodium salts of drugs are avoided.

Initial measurement of water balance while the patient is confined to bed is done by measuring the intake and output of fluid. These measurements are reasonably accurate at this stage but rapidly become less so once the patient is ambulant, when he or the nurses may fail to record the volumes in or out. At this stage a weight chart, the patient being weighed first thing in the morning, then becomes the most accurate measure of fluid balance (Fig. 5.17). The postoperative weight can then be compared with the preoperative figure and diuretic dosage adjusted depending upon preoperative assessment of fluid overload or dehydration. For instance a patient who has been in pulmonary oedema or has had severe tricuspid regurgitation prior to surgery will require a significantly lower weight postoperatively. If the scales used to weigh the patient are different before and after surgery, it is important to know by how much the zero differs between them.

2. *Promotion of a diuresis*
If the urinary output is poor during the first 24 hours, mannitol is useful for promoting a diuresis. Through its osmotic action it reduces absorption of

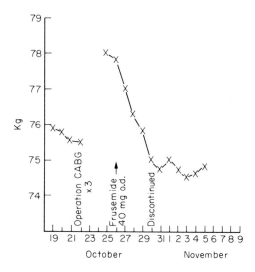

Fig. 5.17. Weight chart of a typical patient having a dilution prime open heart surgical operation. Initial weight gain after surgery controlled with diuretics.

water by the tubules and helps to protect the kidneys from the effects of a low cardiac output. 25–50 ml of a 25% solution are given and the dose is repeated two hours later if it has been ineffective. It is not, however, as effective as other diuretic drugs and in acute renal failure may precipitate pulmonary oedema if given in large doses by drawing water into the vascular compartment from which it cannot be excreted.

Most other diuretics act by preventing sodium absorption in the renal tubules. The increased excretion of sodium is accompanied by water and the extracellular fluid volume falls.

The diuretic that is most effective will change as new drugs are brought onto the market but at the time of writing frusemide (Lasix) is the best diuretic for routine use throughout the postoperative period. 40–80 mg, given once or twice a day orally or intravenously depending on the urgency of the situation, will usually produce the desired diuresis even early in the postoperative period, so long as renal perfusion is adequate. 20 mg given intravenously is used in the immediate postoperative period if the hourly urinary output falls below 30 ml for more than one hour. Potassium loss is inevitable in any diuresis and is replaced routinely. Regular checks are made on the plasma potassium level during any large diuresis, as sharp and unexpected falls may occur in postoperative cardiac patients.

Low sodium fluid retention may occur later in the postoperative period if diuretics have been used to remove sodium but have not been effective in removing an equivalent volume of water. This may be treated by fluid restriction. Spironolactone (Aldactone) is an aldosterone antagonist and tends to retain potassium though promoting a diuresis. It is useful when potassium depletion is a problem. The dose is 100 mg daily in 4 divided doses. Other diuretics (thiazides, etc.) may be useful later in the postoperative period to produce a milder diuresis.

3. *Peritoneal dialysis*
Water intoxication and pulmonary oedema may occur if fluid infusion has been excessive in the presence of oliguria accompanying a reduced cardiac output or acute tubular necrosis of the kidneys. If the kidneys cannot be made to function, the only way to remove the excess water will be by dialysis (page 146).

(vi) LOWERING THE OXYGEN CONSUMPTION OF THE TISSUES
In spite of all measures to improve the cardiac output, it may remain inadequate for tissue oxygenation. Lowering the oxygen consumption of the patient is then essential to allow the vital organs to survive the period of low cardiac output. The venous oxygen saturation will also improve and intrapulmonary shunting have less effect on the arterial oxygen tension.

1. *Sedation*
Anxiety causes restlessness and tachycardia and so raises oxygen consumption. Adequate sedation is used to reduce mental and physical activity to a minimum without depressing respiration unduly. Morphine (omnopon) in small intravenous doses repeated frequently is the best drug for this purpose in the immediate postoperative period, with a tranquillizer such as diazepam (Valium) added, particularly if anxiety is marked.

2. *Artificial ventilation*
Normally the movements of respiration account for 5% of the oxygen consumption of the body, but when the lungs are stiff due to left ventricular failure in a recumbent patient, this figure may rise to 30%. Artificial ventilation has then an important part to play in removing the load of respiratory work and so lowering oxygen consumption.

3. *Prevention of hyperpyrexia*
A raised température increases oxygen consumption. The temperature is therefore kept as near normal as possible with aspirin suppositories, fans, a cooling blanket or tepid sponging. The temperature usually is raised if the cardiac output is low because vasoconstriction of the skin prevents heat loss, and it will fall when the cardiac output improves and vasodilatation occurs. Vasodilating drugs are sometimes used to combat hyperpyrexia (page 77).

4. *Muscular paralysis*
All skeletal muscle activity can be abolished with a muscle relaxant such as

curare or pancuronium. This, combined with artificial ventilation and prevention of hyperpyrexia, reduces oxygen consumption to the lowest possible level in the postoperative period. Muscle relaxants are particularly useful when cerebral damage or poor cerebral perfusion due to the poor cardiac output is causing restlessness or the patient's fighting the ventilator in spite of heavy sedation.

(vii) MECHANICAL ASSISTANCE TO THE CIRCULATION

Once the myocardium fails to maintain a cardiac output that is adequate for perfusion of vital organs in spite of all the preceding measures, death becomes inevitable without mechanical support. There have been many techniques developed to assist the circulation temporarily with mechanical devices to avoid death of the tissues and to remove some of the work load of the heart while it recovers from the trauma of surgery. These devices include diastolic augmentation, counter pulsation (intra-aortic balloon pumping), long term supported bypass, artificial hearts and cardiac transplantation. Only the first is in regular clinical use.

1. *Intra-aortic balloon pumping (IABP)*

Intra-aortic balloon pumping has become accepted universally as the most practical single technique for mechanical assistance to the circulation when all other measures have failed. The balloon is inserted percutaneously or through a Dacron graft sutured to the side of the femoral artery and placed in the descending thoracic and upper abdominal aorta (Fig. 5.18). It is timed from the R wave of the electrocardiograph to be maximally deflated as the aortic valve opens, thereby reducing the afterload and aortic pressure by approximately a fifth and making left ventricular ejection that much easier. When the aortic valve shuts, the balloon is inflated with CO_2, raising the aortic pressure and so increasing blood flow to the coronary, cerebral, hepatic and renal arteries (Fig. 5.19).

The indication for intra-aortic balloon pumping is a patient with a cardiac output so low that he is not expected to survive and yet with a basic haemodynamic situation that would allow long term survival if the acute situation could be overcome. The indications would include patients who would not come off bypass or who deteriorate in the ITU with a cardiac output less than 2 l/min/m² but who have surgically corrected lesions. Contra-indications include sepsis, continued bleeding, aortic regurgitation, abdominal aortic resection and peripheral vascular disease in the legs.

The problems associated with intra-aortic balloon pumping are few but need prompt recognition if the best value is to be obtained from it. If the assist pressure pulse cannot be seen or is small on the arterial pressure base, the catheter is checked for kinks, a chest x-ray taken to check for kinking or malposition of the balloon, more gas is added and the inflation pressure

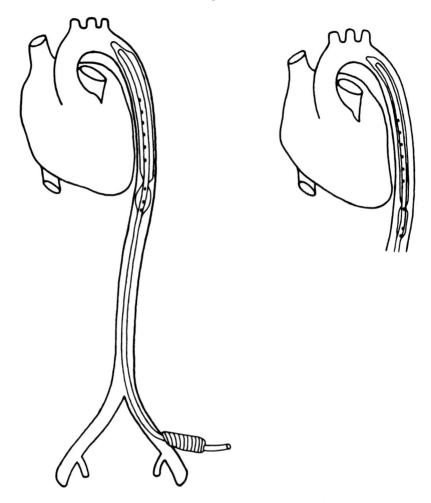

Fig. 5.18. Intra-aortic balloon in position for counterpulsation: inflated in ventricular diastole (left), deflated in ventricular systole (right).

increased in the balloon, and the timing of balloon inflation checked for the appropriate interval after the R wave. Dysrhythmias, such as atrial fibrillation or ventricular extrasystoles, cause irregular assist beats and are managed by intensive treatment for dysrhythmia (page 83) and accelerating the balloon to the fastest ventricular rate, if this is less than 140, or assisting at 2:1 if it is faster. Changing the sensing ECG lead is necessary if the R wave is too small or T wave too tall to permit accurate balloon timing.

The main complications of balloon pumping are leg ischaemia, watched for by absence of the distal pulses, pain or pallor and necessitating transfer

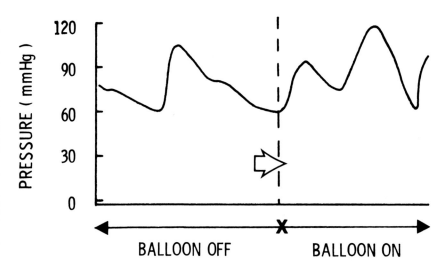

Fig. 5.19. Effect on blood pressure of intra-aortic balloon counterpulsation: increase in systolic and mean arterial pressure. (After Bolooki.)

of the balloon to the other leg; and acute aortic dissection, caused by difficult catheter insertion, which is diagnosed by sudden development of hypotension.

Balloon pumping is discontinued if, after stopping it for four hours, the blood pressure is over 90 mmHg systolic, the left atrial or wedge pressure below 25 mmHg (measured from the sternal angle), urine volume 30 ml/hr and the cardiac index over 2 l/min/m² without massive inotropic support or the presence of dangerous dysrhythmias. It is also usually abandoned if the patient cannot be weaned from it after four days.

2. Cardiac transplantation and artificial hearts
If a suitable donor is available, immediate cardiac transplantation will replace an irreparably damaged heart with another with good myocardial contractility. The chances of having a compatible donor available are necessarily small and an artificial mechanical heart may therefore be the solution of the future. While having been used clinically in the short term, the problems of thrombosis and energy supply have militated against their regular use.

d. DYSRHYTHMIAS

(i) GENERAL MEASURES TO AVOID DYSRHYTHMIAS
The most important measure is adequate preservation of the atrial and ventricular myocardium at the time of surgery. General measures to prevent dysrhythmias include stopping digoxin and diuretics before surgery, giving

adequate—but not more than adequate—potassium during and after surgery and avoiding hypoxia, metabolic and respiratory acidosis and anxiety in the ITU.

1. *Stopping digoxin and diuretics before surgery*

Diuretics cause a loss of potassium so that patients in chronic heart failure may be markedly deficient at the time of surgery, which makes them sensitive to digoxin. Stopping both digoxin and diuretics two to three days before surgery, while preventing recurrence of failure with strict bed rest, helps to avoid this. Fluid retention may occur during this period but this is less important than dehydration and potassium depletion, and the excess fluid will usually be passed during or immediately after the operation when the cardiac output has improved.

It is dangerous to stop diuretic therapy in the presence of severe tricuspid regurgitation because marked fluid overload may occur.

2. *Potassium*

Potassium is given during surgery in amounts which ensure that the patient is returned to the intensive therapy unit with a normal serum potassium. After operation 50–150 mmol are given intravenously each 24 hours in patients who have been on diuretics before surgery.

The exact amount required is assessed by frequent measurements of the plasma level. No more than 13 mmol (1 g) of potassium chloride are set up at one time diluted in 100 ml and given over $\frac{1}{2}$–1 hour. Giving large doses of KCl too rapidly is a common cause of postoperative cardiac arrest and is difficult to correct. While potassium is being given, a watch is therefore kept on the ECG oscilloscope. If the QRS complex begins to widen, potassium infusion is immediately stopped and the serum level checked: if it is high, frusemide (Lasix) is immediately given intravenously. Further rise of potassium is managed as in renal failure (page 144). Some surgeons, including the author, are of the opinion that more postoperative complications are caused by overenthusiastic giving of potassium than are caused by running at a lower than normal plasma level.

3. *Avoidance of hypoxia and anxiety*

All patients are given oxygen by face mask or artificial ventilator to maintain an arterial oxygen tension between 100 and 150 mmHg. If dysrhythmias occur, inadequate oxygenation is looked for by checking oxygen supplies and connections and estimating the arterial oxygen tension.

Anxiety and pain are potent causes of dysrhythmias and are avoided by adequate sedation and analgesia. Anxiety and restlessness associated with ventricular dysrhythmias are treated with heavy sedation or artificial ventilation and anaesthesia with nitrous oxide. This is particularly important after operations for myocardial ischaemia.

(ii) TREATMENT OF SPECIFIC DYSRHYTHMIAS

1. *Bradycardia*
Sinus or nodal bradycardia is treated with atropine, isoprenaline or electrical pacemaking. Sequential pacing via atrial and ventricular pacemaker leads inserted at surgery or later with a P-R interval near normal, may markedly improve the stroke volume in nodal bradycardia. Isoprenaline and pacing are used for the bradycardia of complete heart block. Isoprenaline is given initially intravenously (page 74) and then as Saventrine (30 mg when necessary orally) when intravenous fluids have been discontinued. Temporary pacemaking may have to be replaced by a permanent pacemaker if heart block persists for weeks.

2. *Sinus tachycardia*
Sinus tachycardia is often a sign of a low cardiac output and its occurrence is an indication to look out for one of the causes of a low output. Anxiety, pain, undersedation, CO_2 retention and excessive use of isoprenaline also cause tachycardia. If no cause for the tachycardia can be found and it persists, digoxin may be used to slow the rate somewhat.

3. *Nodal tachycardia*
Nodal tachycardia is difficult to control after cardiac surgery. If it is causing a low cardiac output, it is treated with digoxin unless it could be due to digitalis intoxication.

4. *Atrial flutter and fibrillation*
Atrial flutter and fibrillation occurring for the first time in the postoperative period are best treated by synchronized DC countershock, particularly if they have precipitated a low cardiac output. If they have been present before surgery, recur after defibrillation and are not causing an acute low output state, they are best treated with digoxin (page 75).

5. *Paroxysmal atrial tachycardia with varying block*
This dysrhythmia is most commonly due to overdigitalization. It is distinguished from atrial flutter by the slower atrial rate. Digitalis is stopped and potassium replacement accelerated. Atrial pacing at a rate faster than the spontaneous rate may capture the atria and subsequently slow the rhythm.

6. *Ventricular ectopic beats and ventricular tachycardia*
The serum potassium is checked and intravenous replacement accelerated if necessary. Digoxin is stopped. Lignocaine (1–2 mg/kg initially followed by 1–2 mg/min by continuous intravenous infusion) is added if potassium fails

to control the extrasystoles.* If lignocaine fails to control frequent ventricular premature contractions, disopyramide, quinidine and procaine amide are tried.† Potassium, glucose and insulin solution will sometimes control ventricular ectopic beats when all other drugs have failed. The level of plasma potassium has to be carefully monitored while it is being used. If pacemaker wires have been left in position at the time of surgery, accelerating the heart rate with a pacemaker may abolish ectopic beats.

Ventricular tachycardia requires urgent treatment. The plasma potassium is immediately measured and a low level corrected. Lignocaine (100 mg) is given.* If the blood pressure falls to a low level or the above drugs fail to revert the tachycardia, external DC defibrillation is performed. If ventricular tachycardia recurs on lignocaine, then disopyramide, procaine amide or quinidine are used.

Beta blocking agents (e.g. propranolol) are useful in resistant ventricular tachycardia if it is associated with operations for aortic and pulmonary valve stenosis and a hypertrophied ventricle. It reduces the tone in the outflow tract of the ventricle, lowers the systolic gradient across it and suppresses ventricular dysrhythmias, but may precipitate or aggravate cardiac failure by the removal of sympathetic tone. It has therefore to be used with caution if the ventricular tachycardia has been preceded by poor myocardial function. Beta blocking agents which do not depress myocardial contractility, e.g. practolol (Eraldin) which may still be used in the short term, are preferred if a hypertrophied outflow tract is not a factor.

Preoperative propranolol therapy is usefully continued up to the day of operation before coronary artery surgery but is specifically contra-indicated before correction of Fallot's Tetralogy.

7. *Ventricular fibrillation*
The management of ventricular fibrillation is considered in detail with cardiac arrest in Chapter 14.

e. PULMONARY EMBOLISM

The treatment of pulmonary embolism depends on the size of the embolus,

---

* 400 mg of lignocaine are put in the 100 ml bag of a paediatric Buretrol microdrip set when 15 microdrops per minute ≡ 1 mg of lignocaine per minute. Lignocaine has no significant cardiovascular nor cerebral effects at this dosage level but may cause drowsiness. Confusion and fits may occur if it is given in excessive dosage over days.

† Disopyramide (Rythmodan) is given in 30–50 mg boluses or in a dose of 0.25 mg/min intravenously and increased to 0.5 mg/min to a maximum of 800 mg in 24 hours. The dosage of quinidine, bisulphate or hydrochloride, is 100 mg intravenously slowly over ten minutes and then 100 mg per hour in a continuous drip. Procaine amide is most safely given orally as 1.5 mg daily in divided doses three times a day but can be given intravenously in emergencies where DC shock is inappropriate at a rate of 50 mg/min until the dysrhythmia stops or a total of 800 mg has been given.

the circulatory state of the patient and the length of time after operation that it occurs.

(i) PREVENTION OF PULMONARY EMBOLISM

In the postoperative period after cardiac surgery, there is still controversy as to the best technique of prophylactic anticoagulation. Some units use warfarin, the loading dose being given on the second evening, its magnitude depending on the size, circulatory state and liver function of the patient. 10–15 mg is the usual range. More frequent assessment of the prothrombin time is necessary after cardiac surgery than in ambulant patients as alteration of hepatic function, antibiotic dosage, aspirin therapy and general circulatory state may cause wide fluctuations in response to individual doses. Warfarin is used always if prosthetic valves have been inserted.

Other units swear by subcutaneous heparin during the postoperative hospital stay, 5000 units being given subcutaneously twice a day into the abdomen using 25 000 u/ml strength. The issue is not yet resolved. Pulmonary embolism is fortunately rare after cardiac surgery.

(ii) TREATMENT OF PULMONARY EMBOLISM

1. *Acute massive pulmonary embolism*
Management depends on the degree of circulatory embarrassment.

a. *Causing cardiac arrest or persistent hypotension.* The patient is returned to the operating theatre and emergency bypass equipment prepared for pulmonary embolectomy. Anaesthesia is induced without using vasodilating drugs which may cause catastrophic hypotension in the presence of the low cardiac output associated with the obstructed right ventricle. A median sternotomy incision is made or reopened, catheters inserted into the aortic root and venae cavae, and bypass begun. The pulmonary artery is opened and cleared of clot. The lungs are squeezed manually and by inflation by the anaesthetist to extrude peripheral clot, following which the pulmonary artery is closed and bypass discontinued. The right ventricle may require an extended period of support on bypass in order that it may recover from overdistension. Isoprenaline and digoxin are continued into the postoperative period.

If bypass facilities are not available, a median sternotomy is performed or reopened, both cavae clamped and the pulmonary artery opened, clot removed and a side clamp replaced on the artery within 3 minutes.

b. *With the circulation poor but improving.* A patient who has had an acute massive pulmonary embolus but whose circulatory state, though causing anxiety, is not critical can be treated with intravenous heparin (v. infra) for 2 weeks. Warfarin therapy is begun to maintain anticoagulation when the heparin dosage is scheduled to finish. Streptokinase therapy carries too high a risk of haemorrhage early after cardiac surgery to be a safe therapeutic technique.

c. *With a good circulation.* Treatment is as below (for smaller emboli) if the circulatory state has returned to a satisfactory level.

(iii) SMALLER EMBOLI AND PULMONARY INFARCTION
The treatment of small pulmonary emboli is aimed at preventing a second, larger and fatal embolus. The essential feature of management is the diagnosis and accurate location of thrombus in the veins of the legs.

1. *Anticoagulation*
Anticoagulation with heparin (12 000 u 4-hourly via an indwelling intravenous catheter) is begun. Warfarin is given at the same time and heparin discontinued when the prothrombin time has reached an adequate level.

2. *Phlebography and vein ligation*
The presence of venous thrombosis in the legs and its approximate location are identified with ultrasound or radioactive fibrinogen injection. If these are positive, the veins of the legs and pelvis are outlined by bilateral phlebography, injecting contrast medium into ankle and femoral veins or greater trochanter of the femur. Large recent thrombi identified by phlebography are immobilized by ligating the appropriate veins or removing the clot. If clot is scattered and small in the veins, anticoagulation alone should be adequate.

f. ADRENAL EXHAUSTION

Large doses of hydrocortisone (500 mg 4-hourly) are given. Sodium chloride may be necessary also if the plasma sodium is low.

g. SUMMARY OF MANAGEMENT OF A LOW CARDIAC OUTPUT

The detailed programme of management of a low cardiac output varies considerably between cardiac surgical units and from time to time within these units themselves. A rational programme is outlined here.

When a low cardiac output has been diagnosed, treatment is instituted immediately because the longer it persists, the more difficult it is to correct. The factors to be considered in the management of the individual patient are the filling pressures of the ventricles (preload), the heart rate and rhythm, myocardial contractility, arterial pressure (afterload), oxygen consumption and preservation of other organs.

(i) ADJUST FILLING PRESSURES OF THE VENTRICLES (PRELOAD)

The mean atrial pressure of the ventricle most under stress, either left or right, is raised by transfusion to 12–15 mmHg measured from the sternal angle (15–20 mmHg from mid-chest level). If the right atrial pressure is the higher, the haematocrit (PCV) is frequently checked and adjusted by varying the transfused fluid (page 70). If the higher atrial pressure is the left, the hazard is pulmonary oedema. The bronchi are kept clear of secretions and falling lung compliance treated (page 114).

(ii) EXCLUDE TAMPONADE

At this level of venous pressure, pulsus paradoxus and a dominant systolic descent in the venous wave should appear if tamponade is the cause of the low cardiac output. The chest is then rapidly reopened and clot evacuated.

(iii) ENSURE AN ADEQUATE HEART RATE

With hypovolaemia and tamponade excluded as far as possible, cardiac failure is then the most likely cause of a low cardiac output. If the heart rate falls below 80 per minute, it is raised to about 100 with isoprenaline or a pacemaker. Isoprenaline is preferred if peripheral vasoconstriction is marked, the pacemaker if ventricular ectopic beats are frequent.

(iv) IMPROVE MYOCARDIAL CONTRACTILITY

If the rate is spontaneously faster than 100 per minute, particularly if the rhythm is atrial fibrillation, digoxin is given. The plasma potassium is checked beforehand and digoxin withheld if it is below 4 mmol/l until this has been corrected by giving potassium chloride. If the rate is slower than 100 per minute isoprenaline is infused initially. Adrenaline is used if this fails. Dopamine is indicated when there is tachycardia or poor urine output. If the cardiac output remains low, calcium chloride is given intravenously. The effect of calcium is temporary but is nevertheless of value, particularly if the plasma potassium is high, because the improved contractility may persist. If these drugs fail to raise the cardiac output, glucose and insulin may be tried, again particularly if the plasma potassium level is high (above 5.5 mmol/l).

(v) REDUCE AFTERLOAD ON THE VENTRICLES

Lowering the arterial pressure to reduce the afterload on the left ventricle with vasodilating agents is sometimes of value but may be dangerous if used alone because the blood pressure is usually already low. However reducing the afterload carefully, maintaining the left ventricular filling pressure by transfusion and adding an inotropic drug (isoprenaline, adrenaline, dopamine) will often rescue an otherwise hopeless situation.

(vi) REDUCE OXYGEN CONSUMPTION TO A MINIMUM

If the arterial Po_2 falls, alae nasi move and tachypnoea appears in a spontaneously breathing patient, he is intubated and positive pressure ventilation begun. If he is already on a ventilator, the level of sedation is watched so that anxiety and restlessness are controlled, using muscle relaxants if essential.

(vii) PREVENT EFFECT OF LOW CARDIAC OUTPUT ON OTHER ORGANS

The deleterious effect of the low cardiac output on other organs is reduced as far as possible. Metabolic acidosis is corrected with sodium bicarbonate. If the urine output is below 30 ml/hour ($\frac{1}{2}$ ml/kg body weight/hour), frusemide (Lasix) is given. If this fails in large doses, e.g. up to 500 mg, to produce a diuresis and the arterial Po_2 falls, an additional diuretic or mannitol is given, particularly if the patient has had a dilution prime cardiopulmonary bypass operation. Frequent checks of the plasma potassium are continued if the diuresis becomes brisk.

(viii) ASSESS THE PROGRESS OF THE CARDIAC OUTPUT

Finally, the progress of the cardiac output is carefully monitored so that treatment can be changed or intensified if necessary. Useful indicators for this purpose are the hourly urine output and the level of the temperature gradient in the legs or the toe temperature. In cases of difficulty it is better to measure the cardiac output directly.

REFERENCES

Low Blood Volume

BENTALL H.H., SMITH B., AL OMERI M., MELROSE D.G. & ALLWORK S. (1964) Blood loss after cardiopulmonary bypass. *Lancet* ii, 277.

BERLIN R. (1951) Hyperhaemolysis during the premenstrual period. *J. clin. Path.* 4, 286.

CRADDOCK D.R., LOGAN A. & FADALI A. (1968) Reoperation for haemorrhage following cardiopulmonary bypass. *Brit. J. Surg.* 55, 17.

GARCIA J.B., PAKRASHI B.C., MARY D.A., TANDON R.K. & IONESCU M.I. (1973) Postoperative blood loss after extracorporeal circulation for heart valve surgery. *J. thorac. cardiovasc. Surg.* 65, 487.

GOMES M.M.R. & McGOON D.C. (1970) Bleeding patterns after open heart surgery. *J. thorac. cardiovasc. Surg.* 78, 95.

INGRAM G.I.C. (1961) A suggested schedule for the rapid investigation of acute haemostatic failure. *J. clin. Path.* 14, 356.

KAUL T.K., CROW M.J., RAJAH S.M., DEVERALL P.B. & WATSON D.A. (1979) Heparin administration during extracorporeal circulation, heparin rebound and postoperative bleeding. *J. thorac. cardiovasc. Surg.* 78, 95.

KEDDIE N.C., PROVAN J.L. & AUSTEN W.G. (1966) Central venous pressure, blood volume determinations and the effects of vasoactive drugs in hypovolemic shock. *Surgery,* 60, 427.

MacLEAN L.D. (1964) Venous pressure versus blood volume. *Surg. Gynec. Obstet.* **118**, 594.

McGOWAN G.K. & WALTERS G. (1963) The value of measuring central venous pressure in shock. *Brit. J. Surg.* **50**, 821.

POHLE F.J. (1939) The blood platelet count in relation to the menstrual cycle in normal women. *Amer. J. med. Sci.* **97**, 40.

SMITH B., AL OMERI M., MELROSE D.G., BENTALL H.H. & ALLWORK S. (1964) Blood loss after cardiopulmonary bypass. *Lancet* **ii**, 273.

SPITZER A.G. & BROCK LORD (1968) The recognition of hypovolaemia after open heart surgery. *Guy's Hospital Rep.* **117**, 131.

SYKES M.K. (1963) Venous pressure as a clinical indication of the adequacy of transfusion. *Ann. roy. Coll. Surgeons England,* **33**, 185.

Tamponade

ARONSTAM E.M. & COX W.A. (1966) A new concept of the pericardiotomy syndrome. *J. thorac. cardiovasc. Surg.* **51**, 341.

BRAIMBRIDGE M.V. (1965) Median sternotomy. *Lancet* **i**, 585.

ENGLE M.A., ZABRISKIE J.B., SENTERFIT L.B. & EBERT P.A. (1975) Postpericardiotomy syndrome. *Modern Concepts cardiovasc. Dis.* **44**, 59.

FERNANDO H.A., FRIEDMAN H.S., LAJAM F. & SAKURAI H. (1977) Late cardiac tamponade following open heart surgery: detection by echocardiography. *Ann. thorac. Surg.* **24**, 174.

HARDESTY R.L., THOMPSON M., LERBERG D.B., SIEWERS R.D., O'TOOLE J.D., SALERNI R. & BAHNSON H.T. (1978) Delayed postoperative cardiac tamponade: diagnosis and management. *Ann. thorac. Surg.* **26**, 155.

HILL J.D., JOHNSON D.C., MILLER G.E., KERTH W.J. & GERBODE F. (1969) Latent mediastinal tamponade after open heart surgery. *Arch. Surg. (Chicago)* **99**, 808.

ISAACS J.P., BERGLUND E. & SARNOFF S.J. (1953) Acute cardiac tamponade. Studies by Starling curves. *Fed. proc.* **12**, 72.

KAHN D.R., ERTEL P.Y., MURPHY W.H., KIRSH M.M., VATHAYANON S., STERN A.M. & SLOAN H. (1967) Pathogenesis of the postpericardiotomy syndrome. *J. thorac. cardiovasc. Surg.* **54**, 682.

McCABE J.C., ENGLE M.A. & EBERT P.A. (1974) Chronic pericardial effusion requiring pericardiectomy in the postpericardiotomy syndrome. *J. thorac. cardiovasc. Surg.* **67**, 814.

MERRILL W., DONAHOO J.S., BRAWLEY R.K. & TAYLOR D. (1976) Late cardiac tamponade: a potentially lethal complication of open heart surgery. *J. thorac. cardiovasc. Surg.* **72**, 929.

MORGAN B.C., GUNTHEROTH W.G. & DILLARD D.H. (1966) The effect of blood volume on venous pressure in cardiac tamponade. *J. thorac. cardiovasc. Surg.* **51**, 575.

NELSON R.M., JENSON C.B. & SMOOT W.M. (1969) Pericardial tamponade following open heart surgery. *J. thorac. cardiovasc. Surg.* **58**, 510.

SHARP J.T., BUNNELL I.L., HOLLAND J.F., GRIFFITH J.T. & GREENE D.G. (1960) Hemodynamics during induced cardiac tamponade in man. *Amer. J. Med.* **29**, 640.

SPODICK D.H. (1967) Acute cardiac tamponade. Pathologic physiology, diagnosis and management. *Progress cardiovasc. Dis.* **10**, 64.

VAN DER GELD H. (1964) Antiheart antibodies in the postpericardiotomy and the postmyocardial-infarction syndromes. *Lancet* **ii**, 617.

WERTHEIMER M., BLOOM S. & HUGHES R.K. (1972) Myocardial effects of cardiac tamponade. *Ann. thorac. Surg.* **14**, 494.

YACOUB M.H., CLELAND W.P. & DEAL C.W. (1966) Left atrial tamponade. *Thorax* **21**, 305.

Cardiac Failure

ALPERT J., PARSONNET V., GOLDENKRANZ R.J., BHAKTAN E.K., BRIEF D.K., BRENER B.J., GIELCHINSKY I. & ABEL R.M. (1980) Limb ischemia during intra-aortic balloon pumping. *J. thorac. cardiovasc. Surg.* **72**, 729.

BIXLER T.J., GARDNER T.J., DONAHOO J.S., BRAWLEY R.K., POTTER A. & GOTT V.L. (1978) Improved myocardial performance in postoperative cardiac surgical patients with sodium nitroprusside. *Ann. thorac. Surg.* **25**, 444.

BOLOOKI H. (1977) *Clinical Application of the Intra-aortic Balloon Pump*. Futura, N. York.

BRADLEY R.D. (1977) *Studies in Acute Heart Failure*. Edward Arnold, London.

BRANTHWAITE M.A. & BRADLEY R.D. (1968) Measurement of cardiac output by thermodilution in man. *J. applied Physiol.* **24**, 434.

BRAUNWALD E. (1965) The control of ventricular function in man. *Brit. Heart J.* **27**, 1.

BRISMAN R., PARKS L. & BENSON D. (1967) Pitfalls in the clinical use of central venous pressure. *Arch. Surg. (Chicago)* **95**, 902.

COLTART D.J., CAYEN M.N., STINSON E.B., GOLDMAN R.H., DAVIES R.O. & HARRISON D.C. (1975) Investigation of the safe withdrawal period for propranolol in patients scheduled for open-heart surgery. *Brit. Heart J.* **37**, 1228.

DIETZMAN R.H., ERSEK R.A., LILLEHEI C.W., CASTANEDA A.R. & LILLEHEI R.C. (1969) Low output syndrome: Recognition and treatment. *J. thorac. cardiovasc. Surg.* **57**, 141.

FISHMAN N.H., HUTCHINSON J.C. & ROE B.B. (1966) Controlled atrial hypertension: a method for supporting cardiac output following open-heart surgery. *J. thorac. cardiovasc. Surg.* **57**, 777.

FORDHAM R.M.M. (1965) Hypoxaemia after aortic valve surgery under cardiopulmonary bypass. *Thorax* **20**, 505.

FORDHAM R.M.M. & RESNEKOV L. (1967) Circulatory changes resulting from increasing the venous filling pressure by transfusion following aortic valve homograft replacement. *Cardiovasc. Res.* **1**, 159.

GEHA A.S., SESSLER A.D. & KIRKLIN J.W. (1966) Alveolar-arterial oxygen gradients after open intracardiac surgery. *J. thorac. cardiovasc. Surg.* **51**, 609.

GOLDFARB D. & BAHNSON H.T. (1963) Early and late effects on the heart of small amounts of air in the coronary circulation. *J. thorac. cardiovasc. Surg.* **46**, 368.

HARTZLER G.O., MALONEY J.D., CURTIS J.J. & BARNHORST D.A. (1977) Hemodynamic benefits of atrio-ventricular sequential pacing after cardiac surgery. *Amer. J. Cardiol.* **40**, 232.

HOLLOWAY E.L., STINSON E.B., DERBY G.C. & HARRISON D.C. (1975) Action of drugs in patients early after cardiac surgery. I. Comparison of isoproterenol and dopamine. *Amer. J. Cardiol.* **35**, 656.

JARMOLOWSKI C.R. & POIRIER R.L. (1980) Small bowel infarction complicating intra-aortic balloon counterpulsation via the ascending aorta. *J. thorac. cardiovasc. Surg.* **79**, 735.

KIRKLIN J.W. & RASTELLI G.C. (1967) Low cardiac output after open intracardiac operations. *Progress cardiovasc. Dis.* **10**, 117.

KOUCHOUKOS N.T. & KARP R.B. (1976) Management of the postoperative cardiovascular surgical patient. *Amer. Heart J.* **92**, 513.

LITWAK R.S., KUHN L.A., GADBOYS H.L., LUKBAN S.B. & SAKURAI H. (1968) Support of myocardial performance after open cardiac operations by rate augmentation. *J. thorac. cardiovasc. Surg.* **56**, 484.

MATHEWS H.R., MEADE J.B. & EVANS C.C. (1974) Significance of prolonged peripheral vasoconstriction after open heart surgery. *Thorax* **29**, 343.

MILLER R.R., AWAN N.A., JOYE J.A., MAXWELL K.S., DEMARIA A.N., AMSTERDAM E.A. & MASON D.T. (1977) Combined dopamine and nitroprusside therapy in congestive heart failure. *Circulation* **55**, 881.

PERLROTH M.G. & HARRISON D.C. (1969) Cardiogenic shock: a review. *Clin. pharmacol. Therap.* **10**, 449.

SARIN C.L., YALAV E., CLEMENT A.J. & BRAIMBRIDGE M.V. (1970) The necessity for measurement of left atrial pressure after cardiac valve surgery. *Thorax* **25**, 185.

SARNOFF S.J. & BERGLUND E. (1954) Ventricular Function I. Starling's Law of the heart studied by means of simultaneous right and left ventricular function curves in the dog. *Circulation* **9**, 706.

SEKI S., FUJII H., ITANO T., MURAKAMI T., TERAMOTO S. & SUNADO T. (1974) Regional changes of skin temperature in the leg after open heart surgery. *J. thorac. cardiovasc. Surg.* **68**, 411.

STARLING E.H. (1918) *The Linacre Lecture on the Law of the Heart.* Given at Cambridge 1915. Longman & Green, London.

STURRIDGE M.F., THEYE R.A., FOWLER W.S. & KIRKLIN J.W. (1964) Basal metabolic rate after cardiovascular surgery. *J. thorac. cardiovasc. Surg.* **47**, 298.

WILLIAMS B.T., SANCHO-FORNOS S., CLARKE D.B., ABRAMS L.D. & SCHENK W.G. (1971) Continuous, long term measurement of cardiac output after open-heart surgery. *Ann. Surg.* **174**, 357.

Dysrhythmias

DAVID A.S.M., BROJESH C.P. & IONESCU M.I. (1976) Hemodynamic effects of pacing induced heart rate augmentation. *J. thorac. cardiovasc. Surg.* **71**, 520.

FISCH C. (1973) Relation of electrolyte disturbances to cardiac arrhythmias. *Circulation* **47**, 408.

GUNNING J.F., SHANAHAN M.X. & WINDSOR H.M. (1969) Use of isoprenaline as an antiarrhythmic agent after valve replacement surgery. *Brit. Heart J.* **31**, 83.

HARRIS P.D., MALM J.R., BOWMAN F.O., HOFFMAN B.F., KAISER G.A. & SINGER D.H. (1968) Epicardial pacing to control arrhythmias following cardiac surgery. *Circulation, Supp.* 2, **37** and **38**, 178.

HARRISON D.C., KERBER R.E. & ALDERMAN E.L. (1970) Pharmacodynamics and clinical use of cardiovascular drugs after cardiac surgery. *Amer. J. Cardiol.* **26**, 385.

MATLOFF J.M., WOLFSON S., GORLIN R. & HARKEN D.E. (1968) Control of postcardiac surgical tachycardias with propranolol. *Circulation Supp.* 2, **37**, and **38**, 133.

MURRAY J.A. (1969) Pacemaker therapy for cardiac arrhythmias. *Arch int. Med.* **123**, 355.

ROSE N.R., GLOSSMAN E. & SPENCER F.C. (1975) Arrhythmias following cardiac surgery: relation to serum digoxin level. *Amer. Heart J.* **89**, 288.

SATINSKY J.D., COLLINS J.J. & DALEN J.E. (1974) Conduction defects after cardiac surgery. *Circulation* **49**, 50, Supp. II, 170.

SELMONOSKY C.A. & FLEGE J.B. (1967) The effect of small doses of potassium on postoperative ventricular arrhythmias. *J. thorac. cardiovasc. Surg.* **53**, 349.

SHANAHAN E.A., ANDERSON S.T. & MORRIS K.N. (1969) Effect of modified preoperative, intraoperative and postoperative potassium supplements on the incidence of postoperative ventricular arrhythmias. *J. thorac. cardiovasc. Surg.* **57**, 413.

SMITH R., GROSSMAN W., JOHNSON L., SEGAL H., COLLINS J. & DALEN J. (1972) Arrhythmias following cardiac valve replacement. *Circulation* **45**, 1018.

SPRACKLEN F.H.N., KIMERLING J.J., BESTERMAN E.M.M. & LITCHFIELD J.W. (1968) Use of lignocaine in the treatment of cardiac arrhythmias. *Brit. med. J.* **1**, 89.

WISHEART J.D., WRIGHT J.E.D., ROSENFELDT F.L. & ROSS J.K. (1973) Atrial and ventricular pacing after open heart surgery. *Thorax* **28**, 9.

Pulmonary Embolism

ALPERT J.S., SMITH R.E., OCKENE I.S., ASKENAZI J., DEXTER L. & DALEN J.E. (1975) Treatment of massive pulmonary embolism: the role of pulmonary embolectomy. *Amer. Heart J.* **89**, 413.

BARRACLOUGH M.A. & BRAIMBRIDGE M.V. (1967) Massive pulmonary embolism. *Brit. med. J.* **1**, 217.

BROWSE N.L. & JAMES D.C.O. (1964) Streptokinase and pulmonary embolism. *Lancet* **ii**, 1039.

BROWSE N.L., LEA THOMAS M. & SOLAN M.J. (1967) Management of the source of pulmonary emboli: the value of phlebography. *Brit. med. J.* **2**, 596.

CLARKE D.B. (1968) Pulmonary embolectomy using normothermic venous inflow occlusion. *Thorax* **23**, 131.

COOLEY D.A. & BEALL A.C. (1968) Embolectomy for acute massive pulmonary embolism. *Surg. Gynec. Obstet.* **126**, 805.

GAUTAM H.P. (1968) The surgical treatment of acute massive pulmonary embolism. *Postgrad. med. J.* **44**, 917.

HALL R.J.C., SUTTON G.C. & KERR I.H. (1977) Long term prognosis of treated acute massive pulmonary embolism. *Brit. Heart J.* **39**, 1128.

HIRSH J., HALE G.S., McDONALD I.G., McCARTHY R.A. & PITT A. (1968) Streptokinase therapy in acute major pulmonary embolism: effectiveness and problems. *Brit. med. J.* **2**, 729.

KAKKAR V.V. & RAFTERY E.B. (1970) Selection of patients with pulmonary embolism for thrombolytic therapy. *Lancet* **ii**, 237.

MILLER G.A.H., HALL R.J.C. & PANETH M. (1977) Pulmonary embolectomy, heparin and streptokinase: their place in the treatment of acute massive pulmonary embolism. *Amer. Heart J.* **93**, 568.

SOLOFF L.A. (1963) Postoperative pulmonary embolism. *Amer. J. Cardiol.* **12**, 451.

SUTTON G.C., HALL R.J.C. & KERR I.H. (1977) Critical course and late prognosis of treated subacute massive, acute minor and chronic pulmonary embolism. *Brit. Heart J.* **39**, 1135.

VOSSCHULTE K., STILLER H. & EISENREICH F. (1965) Emergency embolectomy by the transsternal approach in acute pulmonary embolism. *Surgery* **58**, 317.

Adrenal Exhaustion

ALFORD W.C., MEADOR C.K., MIHALEVICH J., BURRUS G.R., GLASSFORD D.M., STONEY W.S. & THOMAS C.S. (1979) Acute adrenal insufficiency following cardiac surgical procedures. *J. thorac. cardiovasc. Surg.* **78**, 489.

CHAPTER 6

Hypertension

Systemic hypertension used to be less often a problem than hypotension after cardiac surgery but the introduction of cold cardioplegia with better myocardial preservation at the time of surgery has markedly increased its incidence. Hypertension increases the afterload of the left ventricle and may precipitate cardiac failure. It also increases the strain on suture lines in the aorta.

1. Aetiology

Moderate and temporary hypertension may occur during the vasoconstrictive phase which may follow immediately on cardiac surgical operations, particularly those involving extracorporeal circulation with hypothermia. Slight and more persistent hypertension follows closure of a persistent ductus arteriosus or aortic valve replacement. Carbon dioxide retention may be associated with hypertension though this is not usually marked after cardiac surgery even when the $PaCO_2$ is considerably raised.

Troublesome hypertension requiring treatment tends to occur in patients with previous essential hypertension, after coarctation resection, or after operations for dissecting aneurysms of the aorta. The hypertension associated with dissecting aneurysms is a critical factor in prognosis and needs particularly intensive treatment.

2. Diagnosis

Diagnosis is simple with a sphygmomanometer cuff or by direct measurement from an artery. The size of the sphygmomanometer cuff should be checked before a diagnosis of hypertension is accepted, as too small a cuff for the size of a patient's arm can cause an artefactual rise of systolic pressure of up to 60 mmHg.

3. Treatment

An abnormally high aortic blood pressure increases the work and hence oxygen consumption of the heart and is therefore undesirable in the immediate postoperative period.

95

a. IMMEDIATE TREATMENT

Management of hypertension involves removal of a predisposing cause such as anxiety, pain, CO_2 retention or hypothermia. Treatment includes posture, sedation and hypotensive drugs. If he is not being ventilated, as after resection of coarctation of the aorta, the patient is sat up at 45°. Heavy sedation with drugs such as morphine may then be sufficient to lower the blood pressure to acceptable levels, but antihypertensive drugs are sometimes necessary in addition, although caution is necessary in previously hypertensive patients, as overenthusiastic treatment may cause critical impairment of renal and cerebral blood flow.

Sodium nitroprusside is made up in solution (p. 77) and given by drip or infusion pump at a rate that reduces the systolic pressure to the desired level. This level is 100–120 mmHg normally, 120–140 mmHg approximately if the patient has been previously hypertensive. Intermittent boluses of phentolamine (Rogitine) may be sufficient (p. 77) for short term control of hypertension.

b. ORAL MANAGEMENT

After reduction of the blood pressure in this way initially, or if immediate action is not essential, oral hypotensive drugs may be used. Prescription of oral hypotensive therapy is best left to the referring cardiologist: new hypotensive drugs are continually coming on to the market and both drug and dosage will depend on the individual physician's preferences.

(i) BETA BLOCKING DRUGS

If myocardial function is satisfactory, as after a coronary bypass graft procedure with a normal ejection fraction, a beta blocking drug such as propranolol (Inderal) will effectively lower the blood pressure. Myocardial contractility and heart rate are reduced so that such drugs are contraindicated in patients with a reduced ejection fraction or if they have bradycardia or a degree of heart block (page 86). They may also exacerbate obstructive airways disease, another contra-indication to their use.

(ii) VASODILATING DRUGS

When beta blocking drugs are contra-indicated, vasodilating drugs, which have no direct action on the heart, are preferable. Hydralazine (Apresoline) relaxes arteriolar smooth muscle and in most patients hypertension can be controlled with less than 200 mg per day. It is inadvisable to exceed this dose because of the risk of provoking a systemic lupus erythematosus-like syndrome. Prazosin (Hypovase) is a useful alternative which, like hydralazine, relaxes vascular smooth muscle. A test dose of 0.5 mg should be given before the full therapeutic dose as occasionally the first dose of prazosin may produce profound hypotension. As it relaxes both venous and arterial smooth muscle, it may be of particular use in controlling hypertension in patients with poor ventricular function.

(iii) COMBINATIONS OF HYPOTENSIVE DRUGS
Moderate hypertension can often be controlled by long acting diuretics, such as thiazides, alone.

The management of hypertension associated with dissecting aneurysms requires special mention as it is probably the rate of rise of pressure (dP/dT) that is important in causing extension of the dissection as much as the level of the mean arterial pressure. A vasodilating drug such as hydralazine or prazosin will lower the mean arterial pressure and is given with a beta blocking drug, such as propranolol, to reduce the force of contraction of the myocardium and blunt the rate of rise of pressure in the aorta.

REFERENCES

APPELBAUM A., BLACKSTONE E.H., KOUCHOUKOS N.T. & KIRKLIN E.J.W. (1975) Effect of afterload reduction on cardiac output in infants after intracardiac surgery. *Circulation* **51 & 52** (Supp. II), 151.
BENZING G., HELMSWORTH J.A., SCHREIBER J.T., LOGGIE J. & KAPLAN S. (1976) Nitroprusside after open heart surgery. *Circulation* **54**, 467.

CHAPTER 7

Blood Gas Tensions and Acid-Base Changes

Alterations in blood gas tensions and acid-base status are an almost inevitable accompaniment of all forms of cardiac surgery, but are most profound in patients whose course has been complicated by prolonged periods of poor tissue perfusion or who have associated pulmonary disease. Changes can occur rapidly and may cause as well as reflect impairment of circulatory function. Frequent monitoring and anticipation or correction of abnormalities is therefore necessary. Monitoring starts soon after the induction of anaesthesia and continues into the postoperative period until both respiratory and cardiac function is stable and adequate.

The results must be rapidly available if they are to be of maximum value, and for this reason the ideal site for the apparatus is immediately adjacent to the operating theatre or intensive care unit.

1. Blood Sampling

Oxygen tension (Po_2), carbon dioxide tension (Pco_2) and pH are measured on samples of heparinized arterial blood, drawn anaerobically. From these are derived the oxygen saturation, bicarbonate concentration [HCO_3] and base excess. The samples are analysed immediately after collection or, if this is impossible, the syringe is stored on ice because the values alter if the sample is stored at room temperature.

Measurements of the mixed venous oxygen saturation in blood drawn from the pulmonary artery are sometimes used as an indirect estimate of cardiac output. As the cardiac output falls, tissue perfusion is reduced and more oxygen must be extracted from each unit of blood if oxygen consumption is to remain unchanged. If however the peripheral circulation is very poor, the blood tends to circulate centrally and little oxygen extraction occurs. For this reason the mixed venous oxygen saturation is a relatively poor index of tissue perfusion.

98

2. Methods of Measurement and Presentation of Results

a. OXYGEN

Oxygen tension (Po_2) is measured directly using a platinum electrode. Oxygen saturation is not commonly measured in postoperative patients but may be measured directly in a haemoreflector.

Po_2 measurement no longer needs skill in maintenance of the oxygen electrode as the assessment is usually made on an automatic blood gas analyser. Some oxygen electrodes may over-read if the patient is on nitrous oxide. The value of measuring oxygen tension rather than saturation is that it provides some assessment of pulmonary function (see Chapter 8) as well as reflecting the adequacy of arterial oxygenation.

b. CARBON DIOXIDE TENSION, BICARBONATE CONCENTRATION AND pH

A short biochemical digression is needed at this point if these three important values are to be understood.

A buffer is the mixture of a weak acid and its salt. It serves to minimise changes in hydrogen ion concentration [H^+] when acid or alkaline substances are added or withdrawn. Although the total buffering capacity of the blood includes haemoglobin, plasma proteins and phosphates as well as bicarbonate, the bicarbonate buffer system is the most important. In this system, pH and carbon dioxide tension are related according to the Henderson-Hasselbalch equation:

$$-\log H^+ = pH = pK + \log \frac{HCO_3^-}{H_2CO_3}$$

which can be rewritten:

$$pH = pK + \log \frac{HCO_3^-}{\alpha Pco_2}$$

where α is the solubility factor for carbon dioxide in plasma.

Two features of this relationship require note; firstly pH is an expression of the reciprocal of hydrogen ion concentration and therefore falls when hydrogen ion concentration (i.e. acidity) increases, and secondly, the relationship between pH and carbon dioxide tension is logarithmic.

There are a number of ways of presenting the relationship between pH, carbon dioxide tension and bicarbonate concentration in graphical form. The pH/bicarbonate diagram (Davenport) is probably the most popular.

In the Davenport diagram, bicarbonate concentration in mmol/l is plotted against pH and the normal state is indicated by the point N in Fig. 7.1a where pH is 7.4 and Pco_2 40 mmHg. A series of carbon dioxide isobars

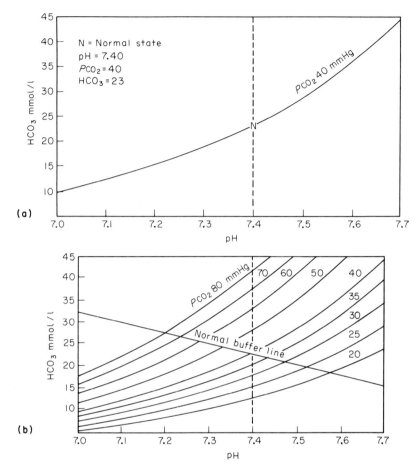

Fig. 7.1. The Davenport pH—bicarbonate diagrams a + b. (Reproduced by permission of Chicago Press).
a. Point N is the normal state.
b. Diagram shows values for pH and bicarbonate concentration at any given level of carbon dioxide tension.

joins the possible values for pH and bicarbonate concentration which fulfil the Henderson–Hasselbalch equation at any given level of carbon dioxide tension. The 'normal buffer line' relates the changes in pH and bicarbonate concentration of otherwise normal blood which is exposed to varying tensions of carbon dioxide. Similar, parallel lines can be drawn to describe the effect of changes in carbon dioxide tension on blood which has a fixed degree of metabolic acidosis or alkalosis (Fig. 7.1b).

It will be seen that the normal buffer line and the isobar $P_{CO_2} = 40$ mmHg divide the diagram into quadrants (Fig. 7.2). Points which fall on these lines

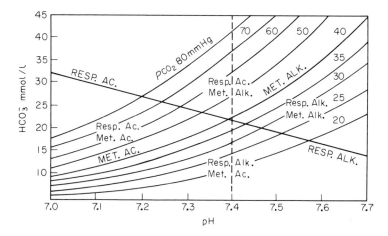

Fig. 7.2. The quadrants of the Davenport diagram which indicate the proportions of respiratory and metabolic changes present.

indicate abnormalities which are either purely respiratory (points lying away from a P_{CO_2} of 40 mm on the normal buffer line), or purely metabolic (points lying away from a pH of 7.4 on the isobar $P_{CO_2} = 40$ mm). Points lying within one of the quadrants indicate mixed disorders which are often the result of compensatory mechanisms tending to restore the pH towards normal, e.g. hyperventilation (respiratory alkalosis) in response to metabolic acidosis. A numerical estimate of the metabolic component of the disorder can be read from the Davenport diagram by measuring, on the bicarbonate scale, the vertical displacement of the point above or below the normal buffer line.

Calculation of the standard bicarbonate ignores the phosphate and protein (mainly haemoglobin) buffers of the blood. All the buffering systems are taken into account by measurement of the *base excess* which is calculated by automatic blood gas analysers from measurements of pH, P_{CO_2} and haemoglobin. The base excess is the number of mmol/l of strong acid or alkali which needs to be added to 1 litre of blood to adjust the pH to normal (7.40 at 37°C and a P_{CO_2} of 40 mmHg). The normal value of base excess is 0. A positive base excess implies a metabolic alkalosis and a negative base excess (base deficit) implies a metabolic acidosis.

3. Indications for Analysis

Information obtained from measurements of blood gas tensions and acid-base status can have both diagnostic and therapeutic significance so that the frequency with which the measurements should be made postoperatively is determined by the clinical condition of the patient. Some of the common abnormalities are given below, together with the probable significance of abnormalities in each case.

a. FOR THE CONTROL AND ASSESSMENT OF INTERMITTENT POSITIVE PRESSURE VENTILATION (IPPV)

(i) AT ESTABLISHMENT OF IPPV

A value for arterial carbon dioxide tension between 30 and 40 mmHg means that IPPV is adequate but not excessive and an arterial oxygen tension between 100 and 200 mmHg ensures full saturation of the arterial blood. Higher oxygen tensions contribute little more to oxygen content and can be undesirable because the greater inspired oxygen concentration required to achieve these levels may cause pulmonary damage.

(ii) FOLLOWING ANY ALTERATION IN INSPIRED MIXTURE OR VENTILATORY VOLUME

The effect on blood gases is checked following any alteration in ventilation or if the ventilator has been changed.

(iii) IF INADEQUATE VENTILATION IS SUSPECTED

(iv) IN THE ASSESSMENT OF LUNG FUNCTION PRIOR TO DISCONTINUATION OF IPPV

A rough estimate of the degree of shunting of pulmonary arterial blood through unventilated or inadequately ventilated alveoli may be obtained by comparing the inspired and arterial oxygen tensions (page 103). Barely adequate arterial oxygenation in spite of a high inspired oxygen concentration implies considerable pulmonary pathology and in these circumstances it is generally wiser to continue IPPV.

(v) TO MONITOR ADEQUACY OF SPONTANEOUS VENTILATION AND OXYGENATION WHEN RESUMED

In the majority of cases, a measurement at this time is only a confirmation of clinical judgement and therefore by no means essential. If there is any doubt about the adequacy of spontaneous ventilation, measurement of arterial gas tensions will be conclusive but it is important to stress that the preservation of normal tensions does not preclude the need to re-establish IPPV in some circumstances, which are considered more fully in Chapter 8.

b. FOR THE ASSESSMENT OF METABOLIC STATE

Assessment of the metabolic state is necessary as it may be both a cause and a consequence of circulatory impairment. Metabolic acidosis commonly develops if there is tissue hypoxia which may be due to defective oxygenation of arterial blood, severe anaemia or a low cardiac output. The acidosis represents the accumulation of lactic and pyruvic acids which are the end products of glycolytic metabolism when there is insufficient oxygen available to complete the stages of the Krebs cycle. Metabolic acidosis also develops in cyanide poisoning from overdosage with nitroprusside.

The return or worsening of peripheral vasoconstriction, a decrease in urinary output, hypotension or a diminishing level of consciousness are all features which may be due to hypoxia (low arterial Po_2) in patients whose myocardial function is impaired. Hypoxia or hypercapnia may provoke dysrhythmias but changes of rhythm can also be precipitated by overventilation, possibly mediated by elevation of the pH and consequent lowering of the plasma potassium concentration.

4. Abnormalities—Their Interpretation and Treatment

a. LOW ARTERIAL Po_2 (hypoxia)

A low arterial Po_2 (hypoxia) is said in practice to be present when the arterial Po_2 is less than 80 mmHg with the patient breathing air. Usually, however, the patient is breathing oxygen-enriched air, in which case the arterial Po_2 should be correspondingly higher.

A low arterial Po_2 following cardiac surgery is more likely to be due to underventilation or pulmonary pathology than to an inadequate concentration of oxygen in the inspired gas mixture. The degree of shunting of pulmonary arterial blood through unventilated or inadequately ventilated alveoli may be roughly estimated by comparing the inspired and arterial oxygen tensions. If this difference is increased, this implies either that the blood is being imperfectly oxygenated in the lungs or that venous blood is passing to the left side of the heart without passing through ventilated lung tissue (intracardiac right to left shunts or pneumonia where there is no ventilation).

Pulmonary pathology which may lead to a low arterial Po_2 includes collapse and consolidation, emphysema, pulmonary congestion or oedema and disorders of the pulmonary vasculature, including pulmonary emboli. Diffuse lung changes may follow cardiopulmonary bypass or transfusion. In these conditions a low Po_2 is largely due to the shunting of blood through totally unventilated alveoli or local imbalance between pulmonary blood flow and alveolar ventilation (ventilation/perfusion or $\dot{V}/\dot{Q}$ mismatch). Arterial hypoxaemia following cardiac surgery is treated by raising the inspired oxygen concentration and by initiating IPPV with, if necessary, a positive endexpiratory pressure (PEEP). Specific measures directed to the cause may also be required (e.g. tracheal toilet and physiotherapy, bronchodilator drugs or diuretic therapy).

b. CARBON DIOXIDE RETENTION (hypercapnia)

Hypercapnia exists when the arterial carbon dioxide tension exceeds 44 mmHg. Acute elevation is associated with a fall in pH (respiratory acidosis) whereas in chronic carbon dioxide retention, the pH is commonly near normal due to the retention of bicarbonate by the kidney (respiratory acidosis partly compensated by metabolic alkalosis). Carbon dioxide retention is always accompanied by a low arterial oxygen tension if the patient is breathing air. If breathing oxygen-enriched air, the arterial oxygen tension may be normal in spite of considerable elevation of the carbon dioxide tension.

Postoperative carbon dioxide retention is generally due to underventilation. Occasionally rebreathing of expired carbon dioxide is responsible if low flow rates of fresh gas are supplied to some patterns of face mask: mild underventilation may also occur in response to metabolic alkalosis.

The conditions listed in the section on hypoxia can occasionally cause carbon dioxide retention, but in the early stages of many of the pulmonary disorders, hyperventilation is more common and results in a normal or lower than normal arterial carbon dioxide tension. Although the arterial oxygen tension in these conditions is always reduced if the patient is breathing air, virtually normal arterial gas tensions may follow the addition of oxygen and it is therefore essential to know the composition of the inspired gas mixture when interpreting the results.

A mild degree of carbon dioxide retention (arterial carbon dioxide tension less than 55 mmHg) is common when the patient has had adequate analgesia with narcotics and is probably tolerable provided it is not prolonged more than 24 hours, the arterial Po_2 is normal and all other systems are functioning adequately, i.e. stable circulation, no dysrhythmias and good urine production. Greater degrees of carbon dioxide retention demand intervention, which generally means a period of IPPV.

c. LOW CARBON DIOXIDE TENSION (hypocapnia)

Hypocapnia (arterial carbon dioxide tension less than 36 mmHg) following cardiac surgery is most commonly due to excessive artificial ventilation. The arterial pH rises as the carbon dioxide tension falls (respiratory alkalosis) and metabolic compensatory mechanisms are slow to occur so that the pH remains elevated.

In spontaneously-breathing patients, a low carbon dioxide tension may be a compensation for a metabolic acidosis (a good example is diabetic ketoacidosis) but is also common in a number of conditions which give rise to hypoxia, e.g. pneumonia, pulmonary embolism and left ventricular failure. Hypocapnia occurs frequently due mainly to hyperventilation in patients with acute circulatory failure even in the absence of metabolic acidosis and if associated hypoxia has been relieved. It may also be seen following some neurological injuries, in association with severe hepatic or renal disorders, and in septicaemia or peritoneal irritation.

The finding of a low carbon dioxide tension in a patient who is breathing spontaneously should therefore be regarded as a warning, and the underlying pathology should be sought and treated. In some patients with left ventricular failure, the paradoxical situation occurs in which hyperventilation is best treated by instituting mechanical ventilation.

In patients already established on IPPV, the finding of a lower than normal carbon dioxide tension does not have the same significance. Mild hyperventilation (arterial carbon dioxide tension 30–40 mmHg) is desirable because it minimises spontaneous respiratory effort and so allows IPPV to be maintained without heavy sedation and with little tendency to 'fight the ventilator'. Even though the arterial $P\text{CO}_2$ is lower than normal, the patient may be best treated by mechanical ventilation in order to improve a low arterial $P\text{O}_2$ by eliminating the oxygen consumption due to the work of breathing. If the ventilator is set so that the patient can trigger it with minimal inspiratory effort, this problem is less. Greater degrees of hyperventilation are probably unnecessary, except in patients with neurological damage when hypocapnia causes constriction of cerebral vessels and reduction of cerebral oedema. Hyperventilation tends to reduce the cardiac output because of an increase in mean intrathoracic pressure.

d. METABOLIC ACIDOSIS (base deficit, negative base excess)

The development of severe degrees of metabolic acidosis was a common problem in the early days of cardiac surgery. Hypothermia, perfusion at low flow rates, inefficient oxygenators, inadequate myocardial preservation and failure to recognize and treat vasoconstriction were all contributory factors. Modern techniques have largely eliminated these problems and it is now rare for a patient to return to the intensive care unit with a metabolic acidosis unless the circulation is inadequate or there has been a period of extreme hypoxia or cardiac arrest.

The underlying cause of the acidosis is tissue hypoxia resulting in the accumulation of lactic and pyruvic acids. Although this is still the most common cause of metabolic acidosis in surgical practice, other conditions such as diabetic ketoacidosis, septicaemia and renal failure are sometimes responsible.

Metabolic acidosis is undesirable. It may impair consciousness, can interfere with the return of spontaneous ventilation, diminishes the effectiveness of sympathomimetic agents and depresses myocardial contractility.

Treatment depends on the cause, the degree of acidosis and the clinical state of the patient. Specific therapy is required for conditions such as diabetic ketoacidosis and renal failure. When tissue hypoxia is the cause, full arterial oxygenation and a normal haemoglobin concentration (i.e. oxygen-carrying capacity) are ensured as far as possible and measures to improve cardiac output and peripheral blood flow may also be needed. These are considered in detail in Chapter 5.

In some patients, a metabolic acidosis may be demonstrable at a time when circulatory function is already improving. Provided the degree of acidosis is not too great (a base deficit of less than 5 mmol/l) it is safe to allow the metabolism of excess acids to occur slowly so that the pH spontaneously returns to normal over the course of a few hours.

If the degree of metabolic acidosis is considerable (base deficit of 8mmol/l or more) or if the clinical condition of the patient gives rise to concern, the pH can be corrected by the administration of sodium bicarbonate. The precise dose required is not always easy to determine because the degree of acidosis is probably varying and the extent of equilibrium between the blood and extracellular fluid may be altered by changes in peripheral blood flow. The optimal dose generally lies within the range

$$\frac{\text{body weight (kg)}}{10} \times \text{base deficit (mmol/l)}$$

to

$$\frac{\text{body weight (kg)}}{3} \times \text{base deficit (mmol/l)}$$

i.e. 70–230 mmol/l for a 70 kg man with a base deficit of 10 mmol/l. The larger dose is most likely to be required if the acidosis has developed slowly, particularly if the causative condition cannot be relieved rapidly. It is safer to give half the calculated dose in the first instance and repeat the estimate of base deficit before giving the second half. If the base deficit is overcorrected, the oxyhaemoglobin dissociation curve is shifted to the left causing impairment of oxygen delivery to the tissues.

Excessive doses of sodium bicarbonate should be avoided because of the large sodium load and the tendency for metabolic alkalosis to develop when the lactic and pyruvic acids are metabolised and bicarbonate excretion is delayed. It is advisable therefore to give a small dose initially, and to repeat this if subsequent measurements demonstrate the persistence of a significant acidosis.

Prolonged periods of cardiac arrest may be associated with extreme degrees of metabolic acidosis, but an arrest which occurs in a patient without previous circulatory impairment can often be corrected rapidly without the development of a serious degree of acidosis. The routine use of sodium bicarbonate in the treatment of cardiac arrest is therefore undesirable.

e. METABOLIC ALKALOSIS (positive base excess)

Mild degrees of metabolic alkalosis are common following cardiac surgery, particularly in patients whose postoperative course is straightforward.

Factors contributing to this include the use of bicarbonate or Ringer-lactate solutions during perfusion, metabolism of citrate in donor blood, potassium depletion, the pre- or postoperative use of diuretics and nasogastric suction. Therapy is rarely required and the condition resolves spontaneously.

Greater degrees of metabolic alkalosis (base excess of 10 mmol/l or more) usually result from the administration of large quantities of sodium bicarbonate during episodes of circulatory inadequacy or arrest. Treatment is rarely required in cardiac surgical patients but may be necessary if the alkalosis is progressive to above pH 7.5. Intravenous hydrochloric acid can be used, an N/10 solution providing 100 mmol/l, but the pH can be reduced more simply by giving cimetidine to reduce loss of H^+ if nasogastric suction is the cause of the severe metabolic alkalosis.

REFERENCES

ALEXANDER S.C. & LASSEN N.A. (1970) Cerebral circulatory response to acute brain damage. *Anesthesiology* **32**, 60.

ASTRUP P. (1956) A simple electrometric technique for the determination of carbon dioxide tension in blood and plasma, total content of carbon dioxide in plasma, and bicarbonate content in separated plasma at a fixed carbon dioxide tension (40 mmHg). *Scandinav. J. clin. Lab. Invest.* **8**, 33.

BROOKS D.K. (1965) Physiological responses produced by changes in acid-base equilibrium following profound hypothermia. *Anaesthesia* **20**, 173.

CARESS D.L., KISSACK A.S., SLORIN A.J. & STUCKEY J.H. (1968) The effect of respiratory and metabolic acidosis on myocardial contractility. *J. thorac. cardiovasc. Surg.* **56**, 571.

KAPPAGODA C.T., DEVERALL P.B., STOKER J.B., PANDAY J. & LINDEN R. (1973) Postoperative alkalemia. *J. thorac. cardiovasc. Surg.* **66**, 305.

MCDOWALL D.G. (1969) Biochemistry of hypoxia: current concepts II. Biochemical derangements associated with hypoxia and their measurement. *Brit. J. Anaesth.* **41**, 251.

MOFFITT E.A., MOLNAR G.D. & McGOON D.C. (1971) Myocardial and body metabolism in fatal cardiogenic shock after valvular replacement. *Circulation* **44**, 237.

MORGAN H.G. (1969) Acid-base balance in blood. *Brit. J. Anaesth.* **41**, 196.

RAISON J.C.A. (1965) Acid-base changes and tissue respiration in extracorporeal circulation. *Ann. roy. Coll. Surg.* **32**, 93.

CHAPTER 8

Respiratory Function

Disturbances of respiratory function occur after any major operation on the thorax. Additional factors may be important after cardiac surgery, including the presence of pre-existing disease of the lungs, airways or pulmonary vasculature, the effect of cardiopulmonary bypass, and the influence of postoperative cardiac failure or neurological damage.

1. Causes of Pulmonary Dysfunction

These additional factors are considered on the basis of the anatomical area affected:

(a) The respiratory centre may have been involved in neurological damage or may be temporarily depressed by sedative or anaesthetic drugs.

(b) The respiratory muscles may be weak due to the residual effect of muscle relaxants, which may be potentiated by antibiotics, e.g. streptomycin and by hypokalaemia.

(c) Pain, wound strapping, chest drainage tubes, collections of air or blood in the pleural cavities or gastric distension in children may interfere with the expansion of the lungs.

(d) Major respiratory obstruction due to faulty position of the jaw or blockage of endotracheal or tracheostomy tubes can be avoided by careful supervision, but insidious obstruction of the smaller air passages due to retained secretions is common. Hyperaemia of the bronchial mucosa and secretion of excess mucus in early left ventricular failure may contribute to this process, which will be worsened by defective humidification or inadequate attention to posture and suction. Diffuse airway obstruction, often irreversible, is common in some forms of chronic cardiac disease, especially mitral stenosis.

(e) Disorders at alveolar level include congestion, oedema or haemorrhage, the ill-defined damage which follows whole body-perfusion—the so-called 'pump lung syndrome'—and chronic fibrosis secondary to prolonged pulmonary hypertension or repeated chest infections. Pronounced differences in regional ventilation are the result. The syndrome of 'high protein pulmonary oedema' may occur within hours of cardiopulmonary bypass. It is characterized by massive outpouring of yellow, protein-rich fluid from the lungs, hypotension, a rise in packed cell volume (haematocrit) and a chest radiograph showing pulmonary oedema.

(f) The pulmonary vasculature may be structurally abnormal in patients with a raised pulmonary vascular resistance when the distribution of pulmonary blood flow is also abnormal. Pulmonary atelectasis and passive pulmonary hypertension caused by a high left atrial pressure produce similar maldistribution.

(g) Age, obesity or the enfeeblement which accompanies chronic cardiac failure may impair ventilation further.

2. Consequences of Pulmonary Dysfunction

The combination of defective ventilation of some alveoli and the maldistribution of pulmonary blood flow leads to mismatch of ventilation and perfusion, resulting in an increase in both physiological dead space and venous admixture. The admixture of venous blood reduces arterial oxygenation even more when the cardiac output is low because of the greater desaturation of the mixed venous blood passing through underventilated alveoli.

Following cardiac surgery the presence of mechanical derangements of the thoracic cage, a high airway resistance and low pulmonary compliance impose a considerable respiratory work load if adequate gaseous exchange is to be maintained Alveolar ventilation is normal or reduced, giving a normal or increased arterial P_{CO_2} with an abnormally low arterial P_{O_2} unless the patient is breathing oxygen-enriched air. This reflects the trivial effect of venous admixture on arterial P_{CO_2} compared with its pronounced effect on arterial P_{O_2}.

The increased respiratory work load may account for a significant proportion of oxygen consumption in the postoperative cardiac patient. This work load, and therefore oxygen consumption, can be reduced by intermittent positive pressure ventilation.

3. Effects of Intermittent Positive Pressure Ventilation

The effects of intermittent positive pressure ventilation (IPPV) on the circulation are mechanical and chemical. The increase in mean intrathoracic pressure reduces venous return. The response of the normal heart is a fall in stroke output especially if there is any impairment of compensatory circulatory reflexes, but when the heart is failing there is less alteration in output following this change in filling pressure. The cardiac output may also be reduced by hypocapnia due to reduction of sympathetic tone on the heart.

Dysrhythmias may be precipitated by positive pressure ventilation if sudden changes in arterial P_{CO_2} or pH are allowed to occur. A raised P_{CO_2} causes a fall in pH and vice versa. Cerebral blood flow also falls if the P_{CO_2} is greatly reduced. Additional disadvantages of IPPV are the hazards of dislodgement or disconnection of the apparatus, a higher incidence of pulmonary sepsis and blockage of the endotracheal tube due to a herniated cuff, kinking or inspissated secretions, particularly with nasotracheal tubes.

Positive pressure ventilation virtually abolishes the metabolic demands of the respiratory muscles and oxygen consumption falls, so that although the cardiac output may also fall, the mixed venous oxygen saturation remains unchanged or may rise. IPPV is also of value in the treatment of pulmonary oedema when the increased intra-alveolar pressure, which may if necessary be maintained during expiration, lowers the left atrial pressure, and so by causing a transfer of blood from the pulmonary vessels to the systemic circulation reduces the venous return. These assets are generally agreed to out-weigh the real or potential hazards of IPPV.

High concentrations of oxygen, up to 100%, can be supplied with mechanical ventilation but may cause further pulmonary damage. However, the systemic hazards of hypoxia are so great that it is generally considered wise to use high concentrations of inspired oxygen if necessary, aiming to keep the arterial P_{O_2} between 100 and 150 mmHg. When the volume of venous admixture is high, some blood will be shunting through totally unventilated lung tissue and will be unaffected therefore by the concentration of inspired oxygen. This means that the increase in arterial P_{O_2} achieved by raising the inspired oxygen concentration may be small, but may be critical in terms of oxygen content over the range of arterial P_{O_2} 45–60 mmHg.

4. Clinical Management

a. TRANSFER TO THE INTENSIVE CARE UNIT

Some idea of whether pulmonary dysfunction is likely to occur in the postoperative period can be obtained before the conclusion of surgery by considering the severity of pre-existing cardio-respiratory disease, the duration and magnitude of the surgical procedure, and the occurrence of transitory or sustained periods of circulatory or respiratory derangement during the operation.

When all these features are favourable—no preoperative disease and relatively minor surgery devoid of complications, e.g. resection of coarctation, ligation of patent ductus arteriosus, closure of secundum ASD—spontaneous ventilation may be re-established in the operating theatre and the patient returned to the intensive care unit breathing oxygen-enriched air from a face mask.

The transition from controlled to spontaneous ventilation, associated with the return of consciousness and the appreciation of pain and anxiety, together with potentially rapid changes in arterial pH, $P\text{CO}_2$ and $P\text{O}_2$, may embarrass circulatory function if this is unstable. To avoid this transition period coinciding with the movement of a relatively unsupervised patient to the intensive care unit, it is wise to continue controlled ventilation at least until the patient is established in the unit and circulatory and respiratory function have been reassessed.

Additional sedation may be required to cover this transition and prevent the semi-conscious, semi-paralysed patient struggling while manual and mechanical ventilation are exchanged.

b. PRINCIPLES OF SETTING UP IPPV

The minute volume required for adequate ventilation is ascertained from the anaesthetist. This minute volume is set on the ventilator with an appropriate rate (10–20) and determines the tidal volume. After connecting the ventilator to the patient, the chest is inspected to confirm that both sides are moving adequately. The appropriate inspired oxygen concentration will have been determined by the anaesthetist.

The arterial $P\text{O}_2$ is regulated between 100–150 mmHg by altering the inspired oxygen concentration and the arterial $P\text{CO}_2$ between 35–40 mmHg by adjusting the minute volume.

If an adequate arterial $P\text{O}_2$ cannot be obtained with an inspired oxygen concentration of 50% (fractional inspired oxygen concentration, $F_1\text{O}_2 = 0.5$), a positive end-expiratory pressure (PEEP) is often applied. This increases the volume of the lungs at the end of expiration (functional residual capacity, FRC) which helps to prevent terminal airway closure and improve gas exchange. It may be dangerous in patients with a low cardiac output due to the raised intrathoracic pressure reducing venous return.

c. SUBSEQUENT MANAGEMENT

The continuation of IPPV for the first few hours of the postoperative period relieves the patient of unnecessary respiratory work and normal arterial gas tensions can be maintained in virtually all cases. During this period, any abnormality of blood volume can be corrected, the rate of continued blood loss assessed and the adequacy and stability of the circulation observed. Estimations of arterial gas tensions will provide some indication of the degree of pulmonary dysfunction if considered in conjunction with the volume and composition of the inspired gas mixture (see Chapter 7).

Final rewarming to a normal or slightly elevated body temperature will occur at this stage. Shivering causes an undesirable increase in oxygen consumption and this can be suppressed with sedation in patients maintained on IPPV without fear of respiratory depression. Body temperature will then rise more slowly but the increase in oxygen consumption will be less.

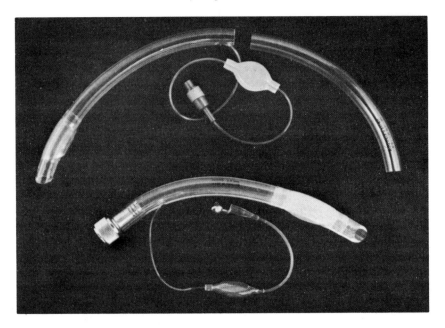

Fig. 8.1. Plastic endotracheal tube. (Above) The tube is cut short prior to insertion into the patient, at the time of operation. The length is assessed with the object of positioning the cuff just below the vocal cords. (Below) The endotracheal tube with Nosworthy connection after removal from the patient.

(i) 'SHORT-TERM' IPPV

It is customary to maintain IPPV through an oral or a nasal endotracheal tube. Plastic tubes are preferred to red rubber because they cause less tissue reaction. High volume low pressure cuffs are used to minimize pressure on the tracheal wall. Ventilation using nitrous oxide (N_2O) may cause a rise in cuff pressure due to diffusion of N_2O into the cuff. A simple manometer is available to monitor cuff pressure.

Plastic endotracheal tubes facilitate this policy because of the low risk of kinking or cuff herniation and the ease of suction compared with red rubber tubes (Fig. 8.1).

The endotracheal tube is positioned so that the cuff lies just below the vocal cords, and the metal connector rests between the teeth rather than in the angle of the mouth (Fig. 8.2). Attention to these points avoids entry of the tube into one or other main bronchus, decreases the risks of obstruction due to biting and prevents painful ulceration of the mouth. The position of the tip of the endotracheal tube is checked on the chest x-ray and should lie 3 cm above the carina.

The ease with which conscious patients will tolerate an oral endotracheal tube varies considerably so that no universally applicable regime for sedation

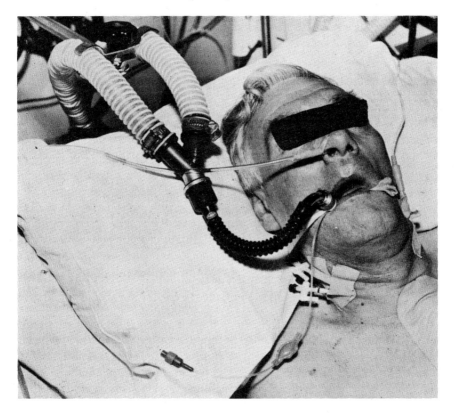

Fig. 8.2. The endotracheal tube is fixed by tape with the metal connection between the teeth and not dragging on the angle of the mouth. A soft rubber tube connects the endotracheal tube to the ventilator tubing, which is supported on an arm to minimise drag on the endotracheal tube.

or management can be recommended. If IPPV is likely to be continued for a few hours only, the analgesic, e.g. omnopon, given to cover the return to the recovery room may be sufficient, supplemented if necessary by 50% nitrous oxide or diazepam (Valium), which has only a slight depressant effect on respiration. By using these agents, adequate analgesia and sedation can be provided while the residual effects of muscle relaxants or narcotic drugs wear off. In this way the patient is optimally prepared to resume effective spontaneous respiration, if judged fit to do so.

Following extubation, humidified oxygen is supplied by a face mask, e.g. 'MC' mask. Oral fluids should be withheld for a few hours as the prolonged presence of an oral endotracheal tube sometimes impairs laryngeal reflexes.

If spontaneous respiration cannot be maintained without undue effort, the signs of distress which occur include:

(1) tachypnoea, often with the use of accessory muscles of respiration and movement of the alae nasi;
(2) peripheral vasoconstriction and sometimes sweating;
(3) a decrease in the rate of urine formation;
(4) clouding of consciousness or restlessness;
(5) hypotension, tachycardia or the development of dysrhythmias.

The classical signs of carbon dioxide retention—hypertension, tachycardia and vasodilatation—are rarely seen.

Measurements of arterial gas tensions following extubation will generally reveal a carbon dioxide tension which is slightly raised and an oxygen tension in excess of 100 mmHg if the patient is breathing oxygen-enriched air. Preservation of near normal gas tensions and often apparently clear lung fields on chest x-ray in no way 'prove' that the patient may be safely left to breathe spontaneously. The decision to reinstitute IPPV is taken on clinical rather than on biochemical evidence.

(ii) 'PROLONGED' IPPV (more than 24 hours)
Many patients can safely resume spontaneous respiration within the first 24 hours after surgery.

IPPV can be maintained satisfactorily through an oral endotracheal tube for at least a week. Tube tolerance can be achieved by careful nursing and the use of sedative or tranquillizing drugs (e.g. morphine, phenoperidine, droperidol or diazepam). During these more prolonged periods of IPPV, efficient sedation, humidification and suction, physiotherapy and attention to posture are required. These points are considered in more detail below. The same care is needed to cover the last few hours before extubation during which the effects of long-acting agents which could depress respiration are allowed to wear off.

Certain patients require mechanical support of ventilation for more than 24 hours. This group includes those with:

(1) severe preoperative pulmonary damage or marked elevation of pulmonary vascular resistance;
(2) a low postoperative cardiac output requiring significant inotropic support;
(3) any evidence of pulmonary oedema particularly 'high protein' pulmonary oedema, when ventilation should be continued for 5–6 days. In the early stages of the latter, adrenaline and steroids will be necessary in addition to counteract the hypotension and immune response;
(4) recent neurological damage.

There are no absolute indications for maintaining IPPV for prolonged periods and each case must be considered individually. The benefits of IPPV must be weighed against the risks, particularly of pulmonary sepsis and mechanical accidents. In equivocal cases, the decision may be influenced by the availability of facilities and experienced personnel on whom the safety of long term IPPV depends.

A short outline of the management of prolonged artificial ventilation is given below.

1. *Choice of airway*
A controversial point is the duration for which an endotracheal tube, oral or nasal, can be safely left in place. Most authors quote a maximum of 7 days but endotracheal tubes can be and are used for much longer periods with no apparent increase in the incidence of laryngeal damage. A tracheostomy is performed after 5–7 days only if it seems likely that IPPV will be necessary for weeks.

2. *Sedation*
Morphine is the most effective sedative drug for use during IPPV. Morphine or papaveretum (Omnopon) may be used alone or their effect enhanced with other respiratory depressants, such as phenoperidine, or tranquillizers, such as diazepam (Valium) or droperidol (Droleptan). The dose should be chosen carefully for each individual taking into consideration his size, hepatic and renal function and the state of the circulation; small doses given intravenously and repeated frequently are preferable to a large 'depot' given intramuscularly. Profound hypotension following intravenous sedation is rare unless the blood volume is inadequate. A slight drop in blood pressure (5–10 mmHg) due to direct relaxation of vascular tone is common and harmless.

The use of muscle relaxants is sometimes necessary if the cardiac output is very low in order to reduce oxygen consumption. Pancuronium is the drug of choice because curare tends to cause a fall in blood pressure or bronchospasm. Although discomfort is probably minimized by the absence of muscle tone, conscious patients may be distressed by total muscular paralysis, particularly if they are not reassured and warned of impending movement or therapy. If the patient is distressed, sedation should not be withheld even if the cardiac output is low and the rate of inotrope infusion has to be increased. The hazards of using relaxants are great and include cerebral damage and death if the ventilator becomes accidentally disconnected with a patient unable to make spontaneous respiratory efforts: difficulty in ensuring adequate sedation of the conscious patient; hyperextension joint injuries; and increased muscle wasting.

The presence of a tracheostomy tube causes less discomfort than an oral endotracheal tube and many patients require no more sedation than would normally be given for postoperative thoracotomy pain. Occasionally, additional sedation is required to depress respiratory effort in patients who attempt to breathe against or 'fight' the ventilator.

3. '*Fighting the ventilator*'

This is usually a sign of underventilation which may be confirmed by measuring the P_{CO_2}. Fighting the ventilator demands a careful examination to determine the cause, which is most commonly a collection of secretions which is relieved by effective suction. Other 'respiratory' causes include leaks in the ventilator circuit or the development of pulmonary pathology, such as collapse, consolidation or pneumothorax. Tension pneumothorax has constantly to be borne in mind in deteriorating patients with high inflation pressures. A sudden deterioration in cardiac output, such as the onset of a dysrhythmia, may initiate fighting the ventilator and any patient with a very low cardiac output is likely to make marked respiratory efforts, often to the further detriment of the circulation. Other causes of fighting the ventilator include pain, distension of the bladder or gastro-intestinal tract, and neurological damage.

If there is no obvious cause for the 'fighting' and the blood gases are satisfactory, sedation is increased. Fighting is less likely to occur if a ventilator with a trigger facility (page 121) is used. Muscle relaxants are avoided unless a reduction in oxygen consumption is necessary to maintain an adequate P_{O_2} or the patient is having uncontrollable fits.

4. *Humidification*

Dry gas supplied directly to an endotracheal or tracheostomy tube will cause drying and crusting of secretions within the airway. Efficient humidification of the inspired gas is essential and can be provided by the passage of the inspiratory gas over a heated water bath so that it is saturated with water vapour. The water bath is maintained at 55°C which prevents bacterial growth in the tank and provides gas which is saturated at approximately body temperature at the end of the ventilator tubing. Modern hot water humidifiers cannot overheat to dangerous temperatures and the only inconvenience of keeping the temperature at 55°C is the increased volume of water condensing in the inspiratory tubing. The best humidifiers have a heated element in the inspiratory tubing which controls the fall in temperature of the inspired gas so that it is at 37°C at the endotracheal tube.

If the sputum is sticky or difficult to aspirate in spite of humidification, normal saline (2 ml in an adult) can be instilled down the tracheostomy tube a few breaths prior to suction.

5. *Suction and physiotherapy*

Secretions within the respiratory tract are removed by suction which must be carried out quickly to avoid hypoxia. Meticulous asepsis is essential. A clean suction catheter, preferably soft and shaped to prevent damage to the mucosa, should be used for each suction and should be handled with a no-touch technique (Fig. 8.3) or with the hands protected by sterile disposable plastic gloves (Fig. 8.4). Maximum efficiency with minimum trauma is

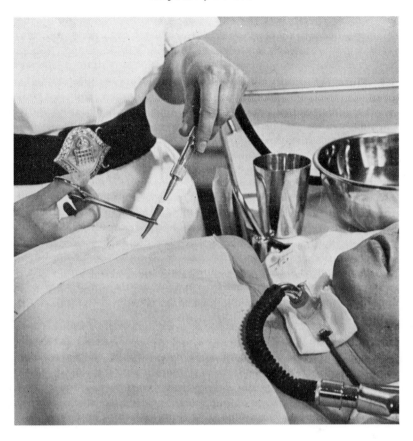

Fig. 8.3. No-touch technique for handling a sterile suction catheter with forceps. Reproduced by courtesy of Dr I.C.W. English.

achieved if the catheter is introduced to the level of the carina while the suction is occluded (Fig. 8.5). Suction is then released and the catheter is withdrawn using a rotatory movement to bring the tip in contact with secretions lying anywhere within the lumen of the trachea or tube. The patient is reinflated immediately after each suction, which is repeated until it is no longer productive. A few breaths of manual hyperinflation before finally reconnecting the patient to the ventilator will help to reverse collapse by the negative pressure.

Suction is carried out 1–4-hourly or as often as necessary. It is convenient to combine this disturbance with change of posture and with physiotherapy. Secretions can be mobilised by the technique of manual hyperinflation with shaking and tapotage (percussion) to the chest during expiration, the 'artificial cough' or 'bag-squeezing' method (Fig. 8.6). Treatment is carried

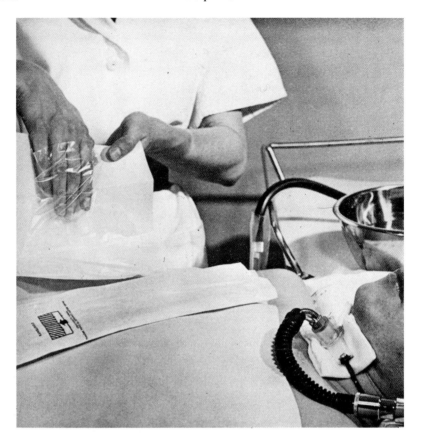

Fig. 8.4. Alternative technique for handling a sterile suction catheter with disposable plastic gloves. Reproduced by courtesy of Dr I.C.W. English.

out with the patient positioned for drainage of first the apices and then the bases of each lung.

If the circulation is unstable, dysrhythmias, hypotension and arterial desaturation may be worsened, but untreated pulmonary collapse can represent a greater hazard.

6. *Nursing care*

Sick patients receiving prolonged IPPV are often immobile and sometimes unable to swallow. Particular care must be given to the skin, eyes, mouth, limbs, bladder and bowels and adequate nutrition should be provided (Chapter 9). A sympathetic and encouraging attitude with full explanation of nursing procedures is of the utmost importance to a conscious, anxious patient.

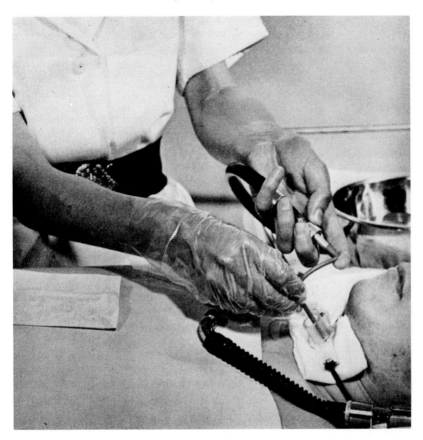

Fig. 8.5. The catheter is introduced to the level of the carina while suction is occluded. Reproduced by courtesy of Dr I.C.W. English.

7. *Discontinuing IPPV*

In ideal circumstances the optimum time to discontinue IPPV is when:

(a) the cardiac output and rhythm are stable and the heart needs little or no inotropic support;

(b) the lungs are clear clinically and on x-ray, sputum volume is small and free from infection, and pleural effusions, if present, have been drained, the arterial blood gases are satisfactory and the inflation pressure is low;

(c) there is no gross impairment of renal or hepatic function. Renal function in particular can be jeopardized if hypoxia is added to an existing renal insult;

(d) neurological function is normal or is not changing acutely because recovery from cerebral damage can be jeopardized by hypoxia or hypercapnia;

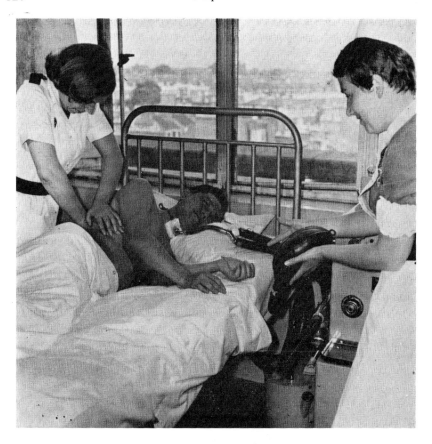

Fig. 8.6. Mobilisation of secretions using the 'artificial cough' or 'bag-squeezing' method. Reproduced by courtesy of Dr I.C.W. English.

If IPPV has been maintained using an endotracheal tube, this is removed when sedation has been allowed to wear off. Subsequent management is described on page 113.

If a tracheostomy has been performed, spontaneous respiration may be re-established gradually, starting with 15–30 minutes at convenient times when the patient is rested. The ritual of 5 minutes in the hour every hour is disturbing and if the patient can breathe for only 5 minutes before showing signs of distress, he is better maintained on continuous IPPV until able to breathe adequately for longer periods. Intermittent mandatory ventilation (IMV) is a useful alternative. The number of breaths delivered by the machine per minute is reduced and the patient allowed to breathe spontaneously to make up the total minute volume. The number of breaths is steadily reduced until the patient is breathing entirely on his own.

Humidified oxygen is provided during the periods of spontaneous respiration using a T-piece. After 24 hours without ventilatory support, the tracheostomy tube may be removed, provided the patient can cough and swallow properly. If there are excessive secretions, a 'speaking tube' (a silver tube with a flap valve on the inner tube) may be useful to permit continued suction. This can be left in place for a day or even longer before final decannulation. Airtight strapping is then applied to the tracheostomy incision and the patient can be instructed to occlude the opening with his finger while coughing or talking.

8. *Choice of ventilator*

Intentionally, this topic has been left until the last because those to whom this book is directed will rarely be in a position to dictate the choice of apparatus. The decision will be influenced not only by clinical considerations but also by the availability of piped gas supplies (particularly compressed air) and whether paediatric cardiac surgery is included. The mechanical requirements of the machine are that it should be capable of providing adequate and preferably constant tidal and minute volumes in spite of high airway resistance and low pulmonary compliance and in spite of variations in these factors. Additional desirable features are:

(a) the ability to change quickly from automatic to manual ventilation;
(b) the provision of a trigger which permits the patient to initiate an immediate inflation by the ventilator when he makes an inspiratory effort;
(c) an intermittent mandatory ventilation (IMV) facility (page 120);
(d) provision for using positive end-expiratory pressures;
(e) ducting of expired air out of the ward area to minimize cross-infection;
(f) acceptable size, cost, simplicity and reliability;
(g) ease of sterilization and servicing;
(h) an alarm if the expired minute volume falls below a preset level.

Most clinicians responsible for automatic ventilation of patients following cardiac surgery prefer a flow-generator with preset volume which is either time-cycled or functions as a minute volume divider. Commonly favoured examples in Great Britain include some models of the Engström, Cape, Servo, Blease and Manley ventilators. The Bird ventilator has the advantage of being cheap and small but suffers from the disadvantages that it cannot produce sufficient pressure to provide an adequate tidal volume in the presence of very stiff lungs and, being pressure-cycled, the tidal volume may fall and ventilation become inadequate if the compliance of the patient's lungs falls (lungs become stiffer). It also often gives dangerously high concentrations of oxygen if it entrains insufficient air when driven by compressed oxygen.

Many other machines can be used successfully, at least in all but the most extreme situations. If the performance of the machine available is fully understood, it can often be adjusted to provide adequate ventilation even if not ideally suited on a theoretical basis to a particular clinical problem.

REFERENCES

ANDERSEN N.B. & GHIA J. (1970) Pulmonary function, cardiac status, and postoperative course in relation to cardiopulmonary bypass. *J. thorac. cardiovasc. Surg.* **59**, 474.

BRANTHWAITE M.A. (1980) *Anaesthesia for Cardiac Surgery.* 2nd edition. Blackwell Scientific Publications, Oxford.

CLEMENT A.J. & HUBSCH S.K. (1968) Chest physiotherapy by the 'bag squeezing' method. *Physiotherapy* **1**, 355.

IVERSON L.J.G., FECKER R.R., FOX H.E. & MAY I.A. (1978) A comparative study of IPPB, the incentive spirometer and blow bottles; the prevention of atelectasis following cardiac surgery. *Ann. thorac. Surg.* **25**, 197.

KAPLAN S.L., SULLIVAN S.F., MALM J.R., BOWMAN F.O. & PAPPER E.M. (1969) Effect of cardiopulmonary bypass on pulmonary diffusing capacity. *J. thorac. cardiovasc. Surg.* **57**, 738.

MIDELL A.I., SKINNER D.B., DeBOER A. & BERMUDEZ G. (1974) A review of pulmonary problems following valve replacement in 100 consecutive patients. *Ann. thorac. Surg.* **18**, 219.

MOFFITT E.A., TARHAN S. & LUNDBORG R.O. (1968) Anesthesia for cardiac surgery: principles and practice. *Anesthesiology* **29**, 1181.

MUSHIN W.W., RENDELL-BAKER L., THOMPSON P.W., & MAPLESON W.W. (1980) *Automatic Ventilation of the Lung.* 3rd edition. Blackwell Scientific Publications, Oxford.

PROVAN J.L., AUSTEN W.G. & SCANNELL J.G. (1966) Respiratory complications after open heart surgery. *J. thorac. cardiovasc. Surg.* **51**, 626.

SINGER M.M., WRIGHT F., STANLEY L.K., ROE B.B. & HAMILTON W.K. (1970) Oxygen toxicity in man. *New England J. Med.* **283**, 1473.

SPALDING J.M.K. & SMITH A.C. (1963) *Clinical Practice and Physiology of Artificial Respiration.* Blackwell Scientific Publications, Oxford.

STEIER M., CHING N., ROBERTS E.B. & NEALON T.F. (1974) Pneumothorax complicating continuous ventilatory support. *J. thorac. cardiovasc. Surg.* **67**, 17.

TRIMBLE A.S. & YORK J.E. (1965) Recognition and management of postoperative respiratory insufficiency. *Surgery* **58**, 765.

CHAPTER 9

Fluid Balance and Parenteral Nutrition

Modern enthusiasm for intravenous fluid therapy has resulted in a tendency to overhydrate many patients. Although this rarely causes serious harm, there are some patients in whom caution is essential and a carefully planned regime of intravenous fluid replacement will be required to prevent dehydration and electrolyte imbalance, without causing circulatory overloading and pulmonary oedema.

In this chapter, sodium and water are considered together and potassium and magnesium balance are discussed separately. In the light of present knowledge, the metabolism of calcium is probably not important following cardiac surgery. Hyperosmolality is rarely of significance in adults but is of critical importance in infants and is considered fully in Chapter 16.

1. Water and Sodium Metabolism

a. NORMAL EXCHANGE

Water balance is achieved when intake and output are equal. Water gain includes the volume ingested plus the volume derived from metabolism. Water loss consists of urine, a small volume lost from the bowel and 'insensible' loss from the lungs and skin. Sodium is derived entirely from the diet and is predominantly excreted in the urine although some is lost from the bowel and through the skin.

Average values for the water and sodium balance of a 70 kg adult under normal conditions of diet, exercise and climate are given in Table 9.1. There is considerable individual variation in sodium exchange and the figures quoted represent a generous allowance. In the Table, sodium and water are expressed as millimoles or millilitres both per kilogram of body weight and per square metre of body surface area. An example is given for a 70 kg man with a surface area of 1.73 m^2. The values have been approximated to whole numbers wherever possible.

123

Table 9.1. Normal daily exchanges for sodium and water

		70 kg man–1.73 m²
1. *WATER*		
Water gain: metabolic water	0.3 l/m² (7 ml/kg)	0.5 l/day
ingested	1.2 l/m² (30 ml/kg)	2.1 l/day
Total water gain	1.5 l/m² (37 ml/kg)	2.6 l/day
Water loss: urine	1.0 l/m² (24 ml/kg)	1.75 l/day
insensible (incl. faecal loss)	0.5 l/m² (12 ml/kg)	0.85 l/day
Total loss	1.5 l/m² (36 ml/kg)	2.6 l/day
2. *SODIUM*		
Sodium exchange	100 mmol/m² (2.5 mmol/kg)	170 mmol/day

b. MODIFICATIONS IMPOSED BY CARDIAC SURGERY

After major surgery, there is a relative inability to excrete a water load and a tendency to retain sodium. Prescriptions for postoperative fluids have to allow for the tendency to retain sodium and water but still provide replacement for abnormal losses.

Additional factors which may complicate the management of cardiac surgical patients include the following:

(i) Heart failure occurring before or after operation will aggravate salt and water retention.

(ii) The preoperative treatment of heart failure with diuretics may have caused dehydration, and diuretics used during or after surgery can lead to further losses of water and electrolytes.

(iii) Haemodilution is commonly employed in priming solutions for extracorporeal circulation apparatus. Some of the additional water is retained following perfusion and is normally excreted in the postoperative period.

(iv) Renal function may be impaired, most commonly due to episodes of prolonged circulatory inadequacy.

'Hidden Transfusion' is a phrase which describes fluid transfused but which can easily remain unrecorded. Transfusions of citrated blood contain 120 ml of acid-citrate-dextrose solution per pint of blood. Fluid is also transfused during the injection of drugs—inotropes, antidysrhythmic drugs and vasodilators are commonly administered in dilute solution by means of a 'drip', although concentrated solutions may be used if an infusion pump is available. Finally, significant volumes of fluid may be transfused when catheter systems for pressure monitoring are flushed. This is common when measurements of venous pressure are made with a saline or dextrose-filled column attached to a centrally-placed intravenous catheter which is also used for the transfusion of blood. Each time a measurement of venous pressure is made, the catheter is flushed with saline or dextrose and considerable volumes of fluid may reach the patient in this way. These sources of additional fluid are particularly important in children or if renal failure is present.

(vi) Artificial ventilation (IPPV) may have complex effects on fluid balance. The release of antidiuretic hormone with consequent water retention may be stimulated by sedative drugs, particularly opiates, which are given to enable the patient to tolerate IPPV. Efficient humidifying devices minimize the insensible loss of water from the respiratory tract and an ultrasonic humidifier can even cause a positive water balance, i.e. gain of water by the patient. Conversely, IPPV can also promote abnormal fluid losses—the presence of an oral endotracheal tube may interfere with swallowing salivary secretions being then removed by suction and a large diuresis may follow the institution of IPPV in patients with heart failure, particularly left ventricular failure.

(vii) Finally, hypoproteinaemia, which is often due to disordered hepatic function, is common in very sick patients with cardiac cachexia, severe tricuspid valve disease or systemic sepsis. Such patients are prone to develop oedema, and renal excretion of salt and water is reduced. Dilution of proteins also occurs with haemodilution primes in the pump oxygenator.

C. RECOMMENDED REGIME FOR WATER AND SODIUM REPLACEMENT

(i) WATER

Many of the factors mentioned in the preceding section predispose to water retention, and metabolic water continues to contribute to the total daily gain. Calculated water loss after cardiac surgery for the first 3 days is less than that inTable 9.1. The basic water prescribed following cardiac surgery on the average postoperative day is usually 800 ml/m²/day, that is approximately 1400 ml in the average adult. This can be given as 5% dextrose intravenously, with reduction in the intravenous infusion as more fluid is taken by mouth. On the day of operation less than the recommended quantities will be required, depending on the volume of fluid administered during the operation and the number of hours remaining in the 24 hour period which is commonly counted from 8 am to 8 am. 500 ml/m² (8–900 ml for the average adult) is usually adequate.

These are basic quantities and additional water may be required to cover abnormal losses from the gastrointestinal tract, skin or kidneys—diarrhoea, high environmental temperatures, sweating or polyuria. Greater restriction may be needed if pulmonary oedema or oliguric renal failure occurs.

If this regime is employed, urine output should be approximately 2/3 of normal, i.e. 16 ml/kg or 700 ml/m²/day. In an average man, this is 1.2 litres in 24 hours or 50 ml/hour. However, urinary output is less predictable than intravenous requirements because renal mechanisms compensate for errors in the estimation of daily requirements and the urine volume varies accordingly. An acceptable minimum urine volume is 0.5 ml/kg/hr (30 ml/hr in an adult). Even if these recommendations are modified to suit individual circumstances, oliguria or electrolyte abnormalities may still occur. The differential diagnosis of oliguria is considered in Chapter 10.

When the patient can leave his bed, the simplest and most accurate guide to the maintenance of water balance is the patient's weight. If the patient is weighed each morning before breakfast, his weight can be charted and compared with the preoperative weight (Fig. 5.17). Dilution primes and the necessity for maintaining abnormally high filling pressures for temporarily failing ventricles frequently cause postoperative weights that are higher than those before surgery. Water intake and diuretic therapy are designed usually to return the patient to his pre-operative weight, but allowance has to be made for the preoperative assessment of the patient who may have been oedematous or over treated with diuretics. The weight is more effective later in the postoperative period than fluid balance charts that are particularly difficult to maintain accurately in ambulant patients.

(ii) SODIUM

Many of the factors predisposing to water retention also cause retention of sodium. A raised plasma sodium concentration (hypernatraemia) may be due to dehydration and haemoconcentration but it also occurs if large doses of concentrated sodium bicarbonate have been given. A low plasma sodium concentration (hyponatraemia) following cardiac surgery is rarely due to sodium depletion or deficiency. Overhydration with salt free solutions in massive dilution pump primes is more commonly responsible but hyponatraemia is also seen in the 'sick cell syndrome' when it may reflect impaired ability to maintain normal ionic gradients across the cell membrane. The use of normal or hypertonic saline to correct hyponatraemia is frequently unsuccessful and sometimes disastrous. This syndrome is best treated with water restriction only.

Greater restriction of sodium than water intake is generally necessary early in the postoperative period and many units give no sodium at all for the first few days. If sodium is given, 1/5 of the daily requirement is adequate. This can best be given by using dextrose 4.3% in saline 0.18% instead of dextrose 5%. 1400 ml then supply 42 mmol of sodium.

2. Potassium Metabolism

a. NORMAL EXCHANGE

Daily potassium exchange in the normal adult is roughly 10 mmol/kg or 40 mmol/m² per day, making a total of 70 mmol in twenty-four hours for the

70 kg man of surface area 1.73 m². Individual variation is less for potassium than for sodium.

Only a small proportion of total body potassium is in the extracellular space (60–75 mmol in the adult) and plasma potassium concentration, which is in equilibrium with extravascular extracellular fluid, is a poor reflection of total body content. This is particularly true of potassium deficiency states where the plasma level is at least partially maintained at the expense of the intracellular potassium concentration. The loss of intracellular potassium is replaced by sodium and hydrogen ions from the extracellular fluid, and this leads to the development of an intracellular acidosis and an extracellular alkalosis. The intracellular acidosis results in the secretion of acid urine, so that the extracellular alkalosis is perpetuated and can only be corrected by the administration of potassium chloride.

b. MODIFICATIONS IMPOSED BY SURGERY

Following surgery, potassium loss in the urine is increased and there may also be abnormal losses from the gastro-intestinal tract. It is often stated that postoperative potassium loss is an inevitable and irreversible component of the metabolic response to surgery. However, it is important to recognize that there are two mechanisms contributing to the loss of cell potassium. Firstly, there is depletion in association with cell breakdown, which is indeed irreversible until anabolism is re-established. This loss occurs in conjunction with that of intracellular protein and water and so lowers total body content, but not the concentration of potassium inside the remaining cells. It is not associated with changes in intra- or extracellular pH. Secondly, there is loss of intracellular potassium secondary to depletion of the extracellular fluid, which is associated with exchange for other cations and consequent alterations of pH as described above. It is this aspect of cellular potassium depletion which can be avoided by the provision of adequate replacement therapy following surgery.

Additional factors may influence potassium balance after cardiac surgery:

(i) Preoperative deficit. Although a considerable decrease in total body potassium can be demonstrated in severe heart disease, this may reflect loss of tissue protein rather than a decrease in intracellular potassium concentration. There may however be selective potassium depletion if diuretics have been used without generous potassium supplements.

(ii) Extracorporeal circulation. Potassium-depleted solutions are commonly employed to prime the perfusion apparatus and this can lead to further potassium loss, particularly if a forced diuresis is established with mannitol or frusemide (Lasix).

(iii) The influence of large blood transfusions. The 'plasma' (i.e. true plasma plus anticoagulant) potassium concentration in stored blood rises with time, but the excess is derived entirely from the cells, there being no potassium in any of the commonly employed anticoagulant solutions. At the date of expiry of stored blood, the 'plasma' potassium concentration may be 30 mmol/l, but this only represents a total of about 11 mmol in a pint of ACD blood (composed of 120 ml acid-citrate-dextrose, 245 ml plasma and 175 ml red cells). The contribution of this free potassium to daily exchange is small unless it is given fast, when the high concentration, as distinct from content, may be significant. In the relatively fresh blood which is generally available for cardiac surgery, the 'plasma' potassium concentration is often normal.

Transfused blood is more likely to influence potassium exchange by alterations in acid-base balance. Stored ACD blood is extremely acid, the low pH being partly respiratory and partly metabolic in origin (see Chapter 7). With rewarming, oxygenation and carbon dioxide release, these abnormalities are rapidly corrected. Metabolism of the citrate anticoagulant then leads to the development of a metabolic alkalosis which causes both a low plasma potassium concentration (hypokalaemia) and an increase in the urinary excretion of potassium. Hypokalaemia is promoted by the migration of potassium ions into the cells in exchange for hydrogen ions, a mechanism which tends to minimize the extracellular alkalosis (buffering function of the cell). The metabolic alkalosis leads initially to the excretion of alkaline urine containing considerable quantities of potassium. Potassium rather than hydrogen ion is exchanged for sodium in the distal renal tubules, a feature which is accentuated by the additional corticosteroid secreted in response to surgical stress. Intracellular potassium concentration eventually falls if this loss is not replaced adequately and the secretion of acid urine then occurs, so perpetuating the biochemical abnormalities. The provision of generous potassium supplements can abolish or minimize all these changes.

c. RECOMMENDED REGIME FOR POTASSIUM REPLACEMENT

There are three reasons for maintaining potassium metabolism as near normal as possible. The ion is intimately connected with the excitability of all forms of muscle, including cardiac muscle; digitalis intoxication can be precipitated by hypokalaemia in an otherwise well-controlled patient, and finally potassium imbalance tends to cause or prolong acid-base abnormalities as outlined above.

It is essential to recognize that ECG changes indicative of high or low plasma potassium levels are late signs; potassium replacement must be based on sensible anticipation of the losses, in conjunction with serial measurements of the concentrations in plasma and urine.

In the majority of patients, potassium loss will be almost exclusively in the urine. For patients with good circulatory and renal function, the provision of 50–100 mmol of potassium daily should avoid reversible potassium depletion (deficiency in excess of that associated with protein loss). It should be supplied intravenously as potassium chloride (1 g KCl contains approximately 13.5 mmol potassium) and infused slowly throughout the twenty-four hour period with frequent checks of the serum potassium.

Provided renal function is adequate, any excess over the metabolic requirements will be excreted so that the plasma level will be maintained within the normal range. If smaller doses are used, plasma levels in the lower half of the normal range are commonly achieved, but may represent the movement of potassium into the extracellular space from the cellular compartment.

d. INCREASED POTASSIUM REQUIREMENTS

The recommended dose of potassium may need to be increased:

(i) If there is a diuresis, particularly if it occurs in response to the use of mannitol or frusemide (Lasix), or the institution of intermittent positive pressure ventilation.

(ii) If the plasma potassium concentration remains low. Ideally a value of 4.5 mmol/l should be achieved. It is the experience of some surgeons, including the author, that maintenance of a higher than normal plasma potassium level is more dangerous than a lower than normal one. A high potassium may indeed reduce the incidence of ventricular extrasystoles in overdigitalized or excitable ventricles, but in a situation where there may be oliguria, low cardiac output, potassium leaving ischaemic tissues or too rapid replacement therapy, levels of 6–8 mmol/l may occur, particularly if frequent potassium estimations have been neglected. This may cause reduced myocardial contractility, widening of the QRS complex and ventricular fibrillation which is particularly difficult to revert, requiring glucose and insulin infusion and prolonged massage. Too low a plasma potassium may cause ventricular extrasystoles and occasionally, though rarely, ventricular fibrillation, but this is easily corrected with 10 mmol of potassium chloride and a DC countershock. A useful regime is to replace potassium with 10 mmols or 1 g intravenously until the plasma potassium is 4.5 mmol/l, checking the level after each 10 mmol infusion.

(iii) In the presence of dysrhythmias, especially ventricular extra-systoles. These are commonly induced by hypokalaemia, even in patients who are not digitalized, and the administration of 5–10 mmol of potassium chloride by slow intravenous injection often abolishes the ectopic beats. The development of paroxysmal atrial tachycardia with block in a digitalized patient may have similar significance.

(iv) When intravenous nutrition is instituted—see page 133.

e. REDUCED POTASSIUM REQUIREMENTS

In some circumstances, the dose of potassium recommended here is too large:

(i) If there is oliguria or if renal function is suspect in spite of a well-maintained urine volume.

(ii) In the presence of a progressive acidosis. This promotes a rise in extracellular potassium concentration, because hydrogen ion is partially buffered by exchange with intracellular potassium.

(iii) If there is evidence of excessive tissue catabolism (e.g. sepsis) or such profound impairment of the circulation that normal ionic gradients across cell membranes cannot be maintained. It is likely that either of these conditions will be associated with impaired renal function and metabolic acidosis. The liberation of intracellular potassium then exceeds the rate at which it can be excreted by the damaged kidneys and the plasma level rises—a situation commonly seen during cardiac arrest.

Any of these features may develop quite suddenly in the postoperative period and prompt adjustment of intravenous potassium therapy may be required to prevent the plasma level rising to toxic levels. This demands frequent reassessment and the constant availability of medical staff authorised to change the regime. For this reason, smaller quantities of potassium are often preferred for routine replacement. The risk of acute hyperkalaemia is thereby lessened, but the possibility of chronic depletion is increased and the development of arrhythmias may be facilitated if the plasma level falls significantly.

3. Magnesium Metabolism

Normal plasma magnesium ranges from 0.7 to 0.9 mmol/l. Magnesium deficiency occurs after open heart surgery, perhaps associated with dilution primes of the heart/lung machine. It gives rise to muscular weakness, lethargy, depression, irritability and fits in children, hallucinations and cardiac dysrhythmias. Associated low calcium levels cause tetany.

Magnesium excess is possible after cardioplegia with large volumes of solutions containing a high magnesium content in small children in whom the solution is allowed to return to the oxygenator. It slows cardiac conduction and at high levels (7.5 mmol/l) causes respiratory paralysis and cardiac arrest.

Plasma magnesium levels are measured if the patient has unexplained cerebral symptoms or resistant ventricular dysrhythmias. Treatment of magnesium deficiency is with intravenous magnesium chloride or oral magnesium sulphate.

4. Calcium Metabolism

Normal plasma calcium is approximately 2.3 mmol/l. Calcitonin plays only a trivial rôle in adults: parathyroid hormone controls the movement of calcium between bone and plasma. Because of the store of calcium in bone, overall calcium metabolism is unlikely to be of significance in the immediate postoperative period after cardiac surgery and total calcium in the plasma does not usually alter significantly.

Calcium is, however, present in the plasma in ionized and non-ionized fractions. The active component is the ionized fraction, which is approximately half the total calcium level depending on the albumin concentration, and which it has been possible to measure simply and accurately only relatively recently and which may vary in the immediate post-bypass and postoperative period, as may the level of parathyroid hormone. Although there is no well-documented evidence that a low ionized calcium level clinically reduces myocardial contractility, calcium chloride (2–5 ml of 10% calcium chloride, 1–2.5 mmol) may be given intravenously in low output states for its temporary inotropic effect. The ionized calcium level may, however, already be higher than normal at these times.

Occasionally in the postoperative period a low calcium level causes tetany but its dangerous clinical manifestation, laryngeal spasm, is rarely seen. A high calcium level paralyses the renal tubules so that thirst and polyuria and eventually coma result: these are extremely rare after cardiac surgery.

Calcium is also necessary in the clotting process (page 170). If citrated bank blood is being given very rapidly, citrate is not metabolized and may bind the calcium. Calcium chloride (1–2 mmol) may be given to cover each bottle of blood transfused. Calcium gluconate is preferred in children because the calcium is not ionized and it is less likely to cause cardiac irritability.

The importance of giving calcium for its effect on both myocardial contractility and the clotting mechanism has been less emphasized in recent years and in many units the use of calcium in the postoperative period is uncommon except in neonates (Chapter 16).

5. Nutrition

Oral feeding is resumed in most patients following cardiac surgery within a few days, and a short period without protein and with only negligible calorie intake is unlikely to be harmful except in patients who are severely cachectic before operation. Attention to postoperative nutrition is important in a small group of patients which includes those who are malnourished, those in whom prolonged coma interferes with the consumption of a normal diet, and those in whom protracted paralytic ileus prevents any form of oral or nasogastric feeding. In this group, the presence or absence of gastrointestinal function dictates whether nasogastric or parenteral nutrition should be employed, the former being preferable whenever possible.

a. NASOGASTRIC FEEDING

If gastrointestinal function is satisfactory, a normal ward diet can be homogenised and injected through a nasogastric tube. Alternatively, nutrition can be maintained with Complan (Glaxo Ltd). This is a powder which mixes easily with water and can be administered through a nasogastric tube; 4 g/kg/day will provide approximately 1.25 g of protein/kg body-weight. The calorie content of this diet may be inadequate, it provides very little sodium and it commonly causes diarrhoea. A modification advocated by Peaston includes additional glucose, sodium chloride if necessary, and small quantities of methyl cellulose. The mixture consist of:

    100 g Complan

    100 g glucose   }   made up to 1 litre

    3 g methyl cellulose

Three litres of this solution daily provide:

    93 g protein

    2550 kcal

    51 mmol sodium

    84 mmol potassium

together with adequate vitamins and minerals. Additional sodium chloride may be added if needed. The urea formed from this high protein intake leads to an osmotic diuresis and water depletion can occur as a result, particularly if there is any defect in renal concentrating power or if water intake is restricted.

A slightly more complex regime, but one that has been found to be more satisfactory at St. Thomas' Hospital, involves mixing 4 tins of Clinifeed 400 with 100 g Maxijul (Carbohydrate) made up to 2000 ml with sterile water in the diet kitchen.

Initially 30ml water are given hourly down to the nasogastric tube and aspirated 4-hourly. If the aspirate is small, a continuous nasogastric feed is given (Table 9.2), starting with half strength and rising to full strength within

Table 9.2. Composition of nasogastric feed: Clinifeed plus Maxijul

Energy	2000 kcal	Vitamin A	1000 µg
Protein	60g	Vitamin D	10.0 µg
Carbohydrate	320 g	Vitamin E	44 mg
Fat	53.6 g	Vitamin B1	1.8 mg
Sodium	42 mmol	Vitamin B2	2.4 mg
Potassium	49.5 mmol	Nicotinic acid	13.2 mg
Chlorides	1000 mg	Calcium pantothenate	6.8 mg
Iron	6.0 mg	Vitamin B6	2.8 mg
Calcium	800 mg	Vitamin B12	19.64 µg
Phosphorus	920 mg	Folic acid	600 µg
Magnesium	156 mg	Biotin	200 µg
Manganese	0.376 mg	Vitamin C	108 mg
Copper	0.752 mg	Sterile water to	2000 ml
Zinc	12.0 mg	Osmolarity	306 mosmol/l

12 hours. 500 ml of feed are dripped in over 6 hours with 2000 ml over 24 hours. Continuous feeds have been found to be preferable to boluses as they cause less diarrhoea: in fact a laxative, such as dorbanex or lactulose, may be necessary in addition.

b. PARENTERAL NUTRITION

A suitable diet for intravenous use is constructed on the basis of normal requirements. Protein should be provided at the rate of at least 1 g/kg body weight/day. Approximately 1/6 by weight of protein is nitrogen and the total calorie requirements may be calculated as 200 kcal/nitrogen. This figure is much greater than the 50 kcal/g of nitrogen required when metabolism is normal, but is necessary to cover the calorie requirements of catabolic patients.

The provision of this total calorie intake can be achieved with a mixture of intravenous fat, carbohydrate and alcohol. It is customary to recommend that not more than 50% of the total calories are supplied as fat and not more than 2 gm fat/kg/day should be given.

With these considerations in mind, an appropriate combination of solutions can be selected. Preparations providing intravenous nitrogen are either protein hydrolysates or mixtures of crystalline amino-acids. The former may contain more sodium than is desirable whereas there is some evidence that the amino-acid solutions may be handled less efficiently than the protein hydrolysates.

Intravenous fat emulsions are the most concentrated source of calories and the soya-bean preparations are probably preferable to those derived from cotton-seed oil. Alcohol is useful as a calorie supplement and is sometimes incorporated into the commercially available nitrogen preparations.

Various carbohydrates are also employed to provide calories. Concentrated solutions of glucose, fructose, and sorbitol are all used for this purpose. Glucose is often poorly handled following surgery and is very irritant to veins. Reactive hypoglycaemia may occur if a concentrated infusion is stopped suddenly, and excessive urinary loss is likely if the rate of infusion exceeds 0.5 g/kg/hour. Fructose is slightly less irritant and may be handled efficiently without insulin. A normal blood glucose concentration will be maintained by hepatic conversion of fructose to glucose so that the brain (which cannot metabolize fructose) remains adequately supplied. Sorbitol is converted in the liver into fructose and is therefore metabolised similarly. It is much less irritant to vein walls than either glucose or fructose, but tends to cause an osmotic diuresis unless given slowly. Up to 10% is lost in the urine when sorbitol is infused at the rate of 0.3 g/kg/hour.

Maximum utilization of the nitrogen will be achieved if plentiful calories are infused simultaneously (e.g. intravenous fat with nitrogen preparation).

Additional electrolytes are generally required, and may be added to everything except the fat emulsion. Apart from the sodium in protein hydrolysates, the electrolyte content of all these solutions is negligible and extra potassium should be provided with the protein (5 mmol/g Nitrogen), and also if large volumes of concentrated carbohydrate are used as the calorie source. An intravenous vitamin preparation should be added to complete daily metabolic requirements.

A caval catheter is frequently necessary to permit the administration of these irritant solutions and the incidence of venous thrombosis is less if the superior vena cava is used. The other complication to be avoided is water depletion. Virtually all the solutions described are hypertonic so that some urinary loss is common and an apparently adequate urine output can mask serious water depletion.

An intravenous regime found to be satisfactory at St. Thomas' Hospital entails giving Vamin with glucose (KabiVitrum) to which is added Addamel for trace elements. In addition 50% glucose with added neutral phosphate and Parentrovite are given.

Table 9.3.

COMPOSITION OF VAMIN WITH GLUCOSE

1000 ml contain:

Energy 2.7 MJ (650 kcal)	Sodium 50 mmol
Water 890 ml	Potassium 20 mmol
Amino-acids 70 g	Calcium 2.5 mmol
Nitrogen 70 g	Magnesium 1.5 mmol
Carbohydrate 100 g	Chloride 55 mmol

AMINO-ACIDS IN VAMIN

Alanine	Lycine
Arginine	Methionine
Aspartic acid	Phenylalanine
Cysteine/cystine	Proline
Glutamic acid	Serine
Glycine	Threonine
Histidine	Tryptophan
Isoleucine	Tyrosine
Leucine	Valine

COMPOSITION OF ADDAMAL

10 ml contain:

Calcium chloride 5 mmol	Copper chloride 5 μmol
Magnesium chloride 1.5 mmol	Sodium fluoride 50 μmol
Iron chloride 50 μmol	Potassium iodide 1 μmol
Zinc chloride 20 μmol	Sorbitol 3 g
Manganese chloride 40 μmol	Sodium hydroxide to pH2.5

Water for injection to 10 ml

40 ml Vamin with glucose are given hourly with 10 ml Addamel added twice a day (Table 9.3). Simultaneously but separately 40 ml of 50% dextrose are given hourly, to which is added 5 ml sodium neutral phosphate over an hour morning and evening with High Potency Parentrovite Nos. 1 and 2 on alternate days (Table 9.4). More dextrose is given if the patient is hypercatabolic.

Table 9.4.

COMPOSITION OF SODIUM NEUTRAL PHOSPHATE

10 ml contain;
Sodium   15.12 mmol
Phosphate   8.53 mmol

COMPOSITION OF PARENTROVITE

Thiamine hydrochloride (vitamin B1) 250 mg	Nicotinamide 160 mg
Riboflavine (vitamin B2) 4 mg	Ascorbic acid (vitamin C) 500 mg
Pyridoxine hydrochloride (vitamin B6) 50 mg	Anhydrous dextrose 1000 mg

---

Hourly Dextrostix tests are done on finger prick blood. A high blood glucose requires intravenous insulin as an infusion at a rate of 2–8 u per hour to keep the glucose within normal limits.

Ideally 500 ml Intralipid (Table 9.5) are given daily in addition to the Vamin. Most patients requiring intravenous feeding are, however, being ventilated and require regular blood gas estimations. The blood of patients on Intralipid (KabiVitrum) clogs up the blood gas analyser and it is not therefore usually given, in the hope that the patient will be able to be transferred to nasogastric feeding within a week. If the patient is curarized, this may not be possible, in which case there is no alternative to giving Intralipid.

A compromise is frequently needed between ideal nutritional therapy and the limitations imposed by other aspects of the patient's condition.

Table 9.5.

COMPOSITION OF INTRALIPID
50 ml contain;
Energy   4.2 MJ (1000 kcal)
Water   375 ml
Carbohydrate   12 g
Fat   106 g
Phosphate   7.5 g

These commonly include the necessity to restrict salt or water intake, and impairment of renal and hepatic function. Renal damage decreases the amount of nitrogen which can be handled, and hepatic malfunction limits the use of protein and fat and possibly also fructose and sorbitol (Chapter 10).

Finally, it must be appreciated that the provision of intravenous nutrition rarely leads to positive nitrogen balance and it is generally impossible to maintain normal plasma protein levels without additional plasma or albumin infusions. It is possible however to minimise unnecessary tissue breakdown, and prevent starvation compounding the underlying pathology.

REFERENCES

ABE T., NAGATA Y., YOSHIOKA K. & IYOMASA Y. (1977) Hypopotassemia following open heart surgery by cardiopulmonary bypass. *J. cardiovasc. Surg.* **18**, 411.

BEATTIE H.W., EVANS G., GARNETT E.S. & WEBBER C.E. (1972) Sustained hypovolemia and extracellular fluid volume expansion following cardiopulmonary bypass. *Surgery*, **71**, 6.

BRENNER W.I., LANSKY Z., ENGELMAN R.M. & STAHL W.M. (1973) Hyperosmolar coma in surgical patients. *Ann. Surg.* **178**, 651.

BRECKENRIDGE I.M., DIGERNESS S.B. & KIRKLIN J.W. (1970) Increased extracellular fluid after open intracardiac operation. *Surg. Gynec. Obst.* **131**, 53.

CHAMBERS D., CHAYEN J., BITENSKY L. & BRAIMBRIDGE M.V. (1981) Ionised calcium and parathyroid hormone after cardiac surgery. In press.

DEANE N. (1966) Kidney and electrolytes. In *Foundations of Clinical Diagnosis and Physiologic Therapy*. Prentice-Hall, Englewood Cliffs, NJ.

DIETER R.A., NEVILLE W.E. & PIFARRÉ R. (1970) Hypokalemia following hemodilution cardio-pulmonary bypass. *Ann. Surg.* **171**, 17.

KHAN R.M.A., HODGE J.S. & BASSETT H.F.M. (1973) Magnesium in open heart surgery. *J. thorac. cardiovasc. Surg.* **66**, 185.

PACIFICO A.D., DIGERNESS S. & KIRKLIN J.W. (1970) Acute alterations of body composition after open intracardiac operations. *Circulation*, **41**, 331.

PEASTON M.J.T. (1967) Maintenance of metabolism during intensive patient care. *Postgrad. med. J.* **43**, 317.

TAYLOR K.M., THOMSON R.M., TURNER M.A., LAWRIE J.D.V. & BAIN W.H. (1978) Hypernatraemic dehydration following tricuspid valve replacement. *J. cardiovasc. Surg.* **19**, 449.

TURNIER E., OSBORN J.A., GERBODE F. & POPPER R.W. (1972) Magnesium and open heart surgery. *J. thorac. cardiovasc. Surg.* **64**, 694.

WALESBY R.K., GOODE A.W. & BENTALL H.H. (1978) Nutritional status of patients undergoing valve replacements by open heart surgery. *Lancet* **i**, 76.

CHAPTER 10

Renal Failure

In the early days of cardiopulmonary bypass, renal failure was often due to inefficient pump oxygenators. Renal failure still occurs but is now most often associated with a low cardiac output and poor myocardial function. It is a very serious complication of cardiac surgery and, even in centres with techniques and staff readily available to provide all types of dialysis, carries a mortality of over 60%.

1. Aetiology

After cardiac surgery renal failure is usually due to acute tubular necrosis (ATN) which is the ultimate result of vasoconstriction. The local mechanisms that cause ATN are not clearly understood but ischaemia may be associated with a physiological shunt that diverts blood from artery to vein depriving the renal tissue of an adequate circulation. Other mechanisms may be involved, including intravascular (glomerular) thrombosis, tubular obstruction and the reninangiotensin system.

Acute tubular necrosis is caused by a low renal blood flow and pulse pressure, both tending to be present together during operative or postoperative hypotension. Incompatible blood transfusion, damage to blood in extracorporeal apparatus, long perfusions, septicaemia, hypoxia and acidosis have also been implicated in cases of renal failure, but tubular necrosis may well have actually been caused by accompanying hypotension. It is a common finding, for instance, that plasma haemoglobin released by red cell trauma after bypass operations can pass through the kidney and appear in the urine without any sign of renal disturbance. Renal embolism with clot, air or antifoam is a rare cause of renal failure, and again may be difficult to dissociate from a hypotensive episode.

2. Pathology

Acute tubular necrosis usually causes oliguria, which is conventionally defined as a urine output of less than 400 ml/day. Anuria, the total cessation of urine production, is rare in acute tubular necrosis and suggests bilateral renal embolism or acute retention of urine due to obstruction at or below the bladder neck (e.g. enlarged prostate). Renal failure due to acute tubular necrosis may occur without oliguria, particularly after valve replacement surgery. This is known as non-oliguric acute renal failure.

Urea and other end products of catabolism accumulate in the blood and the plasma potassium level rises. Other complications are convulsions, bleeding from operation sites or peptic ulcers, nausea and vomiting, an increased susceptibility to infection, and even heart block. In the early phase of recovery from acute tubular necrosis, large volumes of urine may sometimes be passed, particularly if previous fluid restriction has not been adequate.

3. Diagnosis

Renal failure is suspected if there is oliguria of less than 400 ml in 24 hours in an adult, if the blood urea rises or if the urinary urea falls.

Patients with a tendency to develop renal failure will be those in whom renal damage has been diagnosed before surgery or who have had a cause for renal damage during or after surgery. Some patients have frank renal damage before surgery and are accepted with the increased risk of developing renal failure afterwards. Unsuspected renal damage may also be discovered if an abdominal film is taken of the pyelogram that follows injection of contrast medium into the heart or if creatinine clearance studies are performed. During or after surgery renal damage is usually caused by a period of low cardiac output, particularly in patients who already have a low cardiac output due to a raised pulmonary vascular resistance, tricuspid incompetence or myocardial insufficiency.

The patient's records are checked for preoperative renal damage and the operative and postoperative records may reveal a period of hypotension which may have been short but which has been accompanied by a period of low cardiac output and poor renal perfusion before and after the recorded episode.

The essential differential diagnosis is between dehydration causing pre-renal oliguria and acute ischaemic tubular necrosis. The immediate prerequisite is to determine that the patient's filling pressure and inotrope support is optimal to generate the best cardiac output and peripheral circulation, and also to ensure that there are no physical signs of dehydration—dry tongue, diminished skin turgor, reduced eyeball tension (oedema usually excludes the diagnosis of dehydration). At this stage catheterization of the bladder is necessary to exclude bladder neck obstruction, to obtain urine for microscopy and to record the urine flow rate. Once these three objectives have been fulfilled and the differential diagnosis made, the catheter should be removed.

The diagnosis of ischaemic tubular necrosis is supported by a recorded episode of low cardiac output and by the finding of casts and red cells in the urine. If oliguria is present and the urinary specific gravity is less than 1.010, this also suggests renal tubular damage. A specific gravity of over 1.010 is compatible with dehydration but immediately after extracorporeal circulation operations the specific gravity of the urine is an unreliable diagnostic point as it may contain foreign substances such as dextrose or haemoglobin. It is more reliable to compare the osmolality of urine and plasma (U/P). If uraemia is due to extracellular fluid (ECF) depletion alone then, typically, the urinary osmolality exceeds twice that of plasma and, furthermore, urinary urea is high (above 175 mmol/l) and urinary sodium low (below 20 mmol/l) (see Table 10.1).

Some workers have suggested that an intermediate state of 'incipient ATN' may be recognized when, despite correction of the patient's circulatory state, the U/P osmolality remains just above 1.05. They suggest that it is patients in this state of incipient ATN who may respond to intravenous mannitol and frusemide. It is difficult to judge the validity of this concept. It has not been established by controlled trials. However, undoubtedly some patients respond to diuretic therapy after fluid replacement has appeared to be ineffective. The risks of diuretics are small. The administration of mannitol and frusemide is therefore recommended for all such patients. Mannitol induces an osmotic diuresis and may thus prevent cast formation and it may also prevent the swelling of ischaemic cells which would strangle the microcirculation. Its risk is that it may cause a rapid expansion of the blood volume and pulmonary oedema. A single infusion of 25 g (i.e. 50 ml of 50% solution) is unlikely to cause serious problems in the properly monitored patient. Frusemide favourably alters renal haemodynamics, dilating tubules and increasing tubular flow throughout most of the nephron. The deafness it may induce appears to be reversible. The slow intravenous injection of 250 mg has little risk of side effects. Ethacrynic acid is a similar potent diuretic which has gone out of favour in patients with renal failure because of its side effect of irreversible deafness.

Table 10.1. Differential diagnosis of the causes of postoperative oliguria

Cause	Urine			Urine/plasma ratios		
	Micro-scopy	SG	Na(mmol/l)	Osmolality	Urea	Creatinine
Dehydration	Normal	>1.010	<20	>2.0	>14	>20
ATN	Casts and R.B.C.'s	<1.010	>20	<1.05	<14	<20

An oliguric patient with the features of ATN shown in Table 10.1 who has failed to respond to volume replacement and repair of the circulatory state and who remains oliguric following powerful diuretic therapy is diagnosed as having 'established ATN' and managed accordingly. Some patients will have a gratifying increase in urine flow rate following the diuretics but remain in renal failure as evinced by their progressive deterioration in blood chemistry. This is termed 'non-oliguric acute renal failure' and it is an impression that the frequency with which it is encountered has increased with the modern practice of diuretic therapy. Patients with non-oliguric acute renal failure usually have a creatinine clearance of between 5 and 10 ml/min, may require dialysis if hypercatabolic and certainly present a need for careful fluid and electrolyte surveillance. It seems wisest to regard such patients as having a milder form of acute renal failure or one in which the diuretic phase has rapidly supervened (or been induced) on the oliguric phase. The renal histology is indistinguishable from that in patients with oliguric ATN.

4. Prevention

a. DURING SURGERY

Renal failure as a result of operation is prevented by avoiding sudden changes of blood volume due to haemorrhage or inaccurate replacement of blood loss, by providing adequately oxygenated, high flow, extracorporeal perfusion and by maintaining a good cardiac output with the help of drugs such as digoxin, isoprenaline and dopamine.

The kidney tolerates an insult better when it is producing urine than when urine production is scanty. Steps are therefore taken to maintain an adequate urinary output at all times. The patient should not be too dehydrated before operation, either from diuretics or from a prolonged overnight starvation period, nor should he be sent for surgery with the severe dilutional hyponatraemia sometimes induced by potent diuretics. Preparation for surgery must therefore include correction of electrolyte abnormalities and in extreme cases even preparatory dialysis has to be used.

Some 5% dextrose should be given intravenously during the early stages of an operation. The use of osmotic diuretics, such as mannitol (25–50 ml of a 25% solution) given intravenously at a rate sufficient to produce a urinary output of 30 ml/hour, may avert renal troubles from long operations or perfusions. Priming pump oxygenators with largely dextrose or Ringer-lactate has a similar effect. There is no real substitute however for a good cardiac output and an adequate extracorporeal flow throughout the operation. The advent of cardioplegia for myocardial protection has also seen the practice of reducing the extracorporeal flow at 30°C from 2.4 to 1.5 l/min/m^2 of body surface area in order to minimize non-coronary collateral flow from pericardial vessels into the coronary arteries. In the 4 years that this has been the practice at St Thomas' Hospital, there has been no change in bicarbonate requirement nor rise in the incidence of postoperative cerebral or renal problems.

b. IN THE POSTOPERATIVE PERIOD

A low cardiac output in the postoperative period for any of the reasons outlined in Chapter 5 can cause renal failure and every effort is made to keep the blood volume optimal, the cardiac output adequate and the systolic blood pressure above 90 mmHg. If, in spite of these measures, the urine flow falls below 30 ml per hour (0.5 ml/g per hour), frusemide is then given. Mannitol in a dose of 25–50 ml may be given but if urine production does not rise after a second dose 2 hours later, it is not repeated as attraction of water into the circulation may further embarrass an already failing heart.

Achievement of the optimum circulatory state in the postoperative period may require a high CVP and, depending upon the relationship between right and left sided filling pressures, there is a risk of causing pulmonary oedema in an oliguric patient. An intensive care unit fully equipped with dialysis techniques can cope with this situation by performing an ultrafiltration to remove plasma water. This technique is a useful support when adjusting the circulatory dynamics in patients in whom the dividing line between adequate and excessive filling pressure is a fine one.

5. Treatment of Renal Failure

a. ROLE OF DIALYSIS

Once the diagnosis of established ATN has been made, we do not advise playing brinkmanship with uraemia as once tended to happen. There is nothing to be gained from waiting for a critical sign or symptom or biochemical measurement before starting dialysis. Nowadays dialysis can be accomplished with little risk. Moreover, dialysis makes it possible to improve other aspects of the management of these dangerously ill patients. It is often begun in order to help in making adjustments to the patient's fluid volumes and filling pressures. Plasma water can be removed and replaced by blood or plasma. A planned regular dialysis schedule makes it possible to feed the patient. Intravenous or nasogastric feeding is often critical to these patients whose nutritional status largely determines their ability to combat potentially lethal infections. It follows that dialysis should be instituted early rather than late. Some authors have called this modern approach 'prophylactic dialysis'.

To summarize the role of dialysis in the management of the postoperative patient with renal failure, dialysis is used:

(i) To control the metabolic changes, measured and unidentified, which accompany uraemia. The rate of biochemical changes dictates the frequency and efficiency of dialysis.

(ii) To correct the fluid balance and circulatory dynamics in order to achieve optimum cardiac output and to prevent pulmonary oedema.

(iii) To permit the administration of a high calorie, high essential amino acid feeding routine.

b. GENERAL PRINCIPLES OF MANAGEMENT

Enlightened use of modern dialysis techniques does not obviate the need to follow good conservative principles of care of the patient with renal failure.

The natural history of acute tubular necrosis has been well documented. The length of the oliguric phase varies widely but averages around 11 days. If oliguria persists beyond 4 weeks there is a growing likelihood that the underlying lesion is cortical necrosis and recovery becomes progressively less likely. The oliguric phase is followed by the diuretic phase which is conventionally subdivided into the early diuretic phase when the blood urea does not fall spontaneously and the late diuretic phase when progressive increase in glomerular filtration rate occurs. In the early diuretic phase, glomerular filtration rate is low despite copious urine and dialysis may still be required, especially if the patient is catabolic. The ready availability of dialysis has obscured the dividing lines between the phases of the illness, but biochemical results indicate when renal function is recovering and the only risk of going on longer with dialysis is the risk of hypotension due to hypovolaemia. The volume of dilute urine passed during the diuretic phase is to some extent influenced by the state of hydration of the patient at the end of the oliguric phase, but there is no doubt that occasional patients can become depleted of sodium and water and of potassium during the diuretic phase. It is therefore recommended that oral supplements of sodium and potassium are administered and progressively withdrawn from the 10th day of the diuretic phase when most patients can conserve sodium efficiently.

Nowadays, death in patients who develop renal failure after cardiac surgery is not due to uraemia. A cascade of problems develops including septicaemia, pneumonia, gastrointestinal tract haemorrhage, jaundice and hepatic failure, complications of the surgical procedure and, most critically, prolonged low cardiac output. This remorseless march of events in the ITU has been aptly named 'Sequential System Failure'. The experienced team will recognize it and withdraw inappropriate supportive treatment such as dialysis when it is no longer justified.

c. SPECIAL POINTS IN THE CARE OF THE PATIENTS WITH RENAL FAILURE

(i) CONTROL OF FLUID STATUS

Water overloading is always a danger in the oliguric patient but all these patients will have CVP and arterial pressure monitoring, and early warning should be given of the risk of pulmonary oedema. If it is possible to monitor body weight, this is very helpful because of the variability of insensible fluid losses especially in the ventilated air conditioned environments of intensive care. The catabolic patient with renal failure may lose 0.5–1.0 kg body weight per day. It is necessary to permit this weight loss in order to avoid fluid overload. Hypervolaemia very occasionally requires venesection.

Ultrafiltration (without dialysis) removes plasma water without causing any change in the osmolality of the blood. In this technique the blood is passed through a haemodialyser with a high pressure on the blood compartment and without dialysis fluid being circulated through the dialyser. The rate of ultrafiltration can be measured by special devices or, alternatively, plasma water is collected in a measuring cylinder. When fluid is removed in this way it has much less effect on circulatory dynamics than when it is removed during dialysis. Thus, hypotension, nausea and muscle cramps occur less frequently. It is possible to remove 1–2 litres of fluid per hour and dramatically improve the condition of a patient who has pulmonary oedema. This technique can be used in any patient with cardiac failure who does not respond to diuretics. It is normally employed in conjunction with haemodialysis as sequential treatment, the ultrafiltration being done either before or after the dialysis.

(ii) FEEDING REGIMES

The purpose of an aggressive feeding policy in these patients is to inhibit protein breakdown and to maintain good nutritional status and resistance to infection.

Uraemia is delayed by inhibiting protein breakdown. Urea is an end product of protein catabolism, as almost certainly are other products so far unidentified that are more toxic than urea. Some body protein is broken down in the postoperative period in spite of any steps taken but breakdown to provide energy can be limited by supplying carbohydrate as a protein sparer. In the early days of postoperative renal failure the mainstay will be 50% glucose solution administered via a central vein and covered with an infusion of insulin. The rate of insulin infusion can be simply monitored using Dextrostix and an Ames' reflectance meter at the bedside but biochemical determination of blood sugar is usually available in an intensive care ward. Fructose and sorbitol infusions and alcohol, fat and amino-acid infusions have also been recommended. It is seldom possible to achieve the target of 70 kcal/kg body weight. Intravenous amino-acids and vitamin supplements are often given over the last hour of each haemodialysis session. These supplements are especially necessary when patients are receiving dialysis because they are removed from the blood during dialysis. Intensive parenteral 'hyperalimentation' requires careful monitoring of all electrolytes including phosphate which is not present in dialysis solutions. Hypophos-

phataemia is a frequently overlooked cause of neuromuscular and haematological complications.

Oral feeding should be resumed as soon as possible and a period of
nasogastric tube feeding may be valuable. Hypertonic tube feeds cause
diarrhoea and the removal of fluid by dialysis is important in facilitating oral
feeding as well as for parenteral nutrition. It is found that the osmolality of
the tube feed can be increased slowly over several days. Egg and Portagen
(Mead Johnson) are used as the main protein sources at St. Thomas' Hospital.
Portagen is free of lactose, to which some patients are sensitive. It contains
MCT (medium chain triglycerides) oil, which is easily hydrolysed, and corn
oil for energy and the essential amino acid, linoleic acid, and is fortified with
vitamins and minerals. Caloreen (Roussel) is used to supply energy. It is a
glucose polymer and is used in preference to mono- or disaccharides to
reduce osmolality.

With modern emphasis on prophylactic daily haemodialysis and
aggressive feeding regimes, the use of anabolic steroids in an attempt to
reverse the postoperative protein catabolic phase is irrelevant.

(iii) CONTROL OF SERUM POTASSIUM

During the early phase of renal failure it is important to prevent rises in
plasma potassium. Hyperkalaemia causes a sequence of ECG changes—
'tenting' of the T waves, loss of P waves, broadening of the QRS complex,
ventricular tachycardia and, eventually, ventricular fibrillation. Rising
plasma potassium can be controlled by reduction of intake, by ion exchange
resins and by giving glucose and insulin. Potassium intake is reduced to a
minimum in the diet, and no drugs containing potassium are given.

Ion exchange resins remove potassium from the extracellular space into
the bowel in exchange for another kation. 15 g of calcium resonium (Zeokarb)
are given 6-hourly by mouth in as little water as possible. The mixture is
granular and unpalatable but patients can be taught to tolerate it or it can be
given by gastric tube. Resonium A, another ion exchange resin, donates
sodium in exchange for the potassium it extracts, which is undesirable after
cardiac surgery. Calcium resonium donates calcium and is therefore
preferable to Resonium A. If oral intake is impossible, 30 g calcium resonium
may be given 6-hourly per rectum.

Ion exchange resins act relatively slowly and a quicker method is
sometimes necessary. If the serum potassium has been allowed to rise above
7 mmol/l or cardiac complications are occurring, a caval catheter is inserted
and 50% dextrose containing 50 u of insulin per 500 ml is infused
intravenously. 100–200 ml are usually necessary to reduce the plasma
potassium below 6 mmol/l, potassium being driven back into the cells, so
gaining time for the ion exchange resins to act. Frequent potassium
estimations are necessary in order to judge when to stop the infusion, but
correction of the ECG changes of hyperkalaemia occurs promptly.

Once dialysis has been initiated care must be taken to avoid falls in plasma potassium, especially in digitalized patients. Both prophylactic daily haemodialysis and continuous peritoneal dialysis can be safely performed with a dialysis fluid potassium concentration of 4 mmol/l.

(iv) PREVENTION OF DRUG TOXICITY

Any drug which is normally excreted by the kidney must be given in a modified regime in any patient with renal failure. Thus digoxin and certain antibiotics, amino-glycosides, vancomycin and cephalosporins must be administered in reduced dosage. The rule is that it is always safe to give a normal loading dose: subsequent maintenance doses must either be reduced in size or frequency because of the prolonged serum half life of these drugs. If, for instance, gentamicin is required for a gram negative septicaemia, it is preferable to monitor its dosage with blood levels. Other drugs, for instance penicillin and erythromycin which are excreted by the liver, may be given in normal schedules but if one is about to administer an antibiotic to a patient with renal failure—think!

(d) HAEMODIALYSIS OR PERITONEAL DIALYSIS?

Peritoneal dialysis is the first choice. The patient does not need to be moved to a specialized unit because the method is simple and the equipment is readily available and takes up little space. The patient is not heparinized and vascular access does not have to be created. Fluid shifts occur slowly and can be handled by the regular team responsible for care of the postoperative cardiac patient. It is particularly suitable for small children.

However, peritoneal dialysis has its shortcomings. It cannot be used if the diaphragm or the retroperitoneal space has been opened by the surgeon. If there is a surgical or congenital aperture in the diaphragm the pleural space fills with the peritoneal dialysis fluid. If the retroperitoneal space has been opened, the introduction of infection into this space is a serious hazard. Peritonitis is a serious complication which sometimes responds promptly to the addition of an antibiotic to the dialysis fluid but not infrequently limits the efficiency and comfort of the procedure and forces the change to haemodialysis. Peritoneal dialysis is four to six times slower than haemodialysis in correcting biochemical abnormalities (Fig. 10.1). This is a disadvantage if the patient is hypercatabolic (blood urea rising more than 10 mmol/l or 60 mg/100 ml per 24 hours) in which case peritoneal dialysis may not be sufficient to control the biochemical changes. From a nutritional point of view, although losses of amino-acids are approximately the same for continuous peritoneal dialysis and daily haemodialysis, peritoneal dialysis incurs further loss of 20–40 g protein per day. Furthermore, the use of hypertonic peritoneal solutions to remove fluid is not always precise and predictable and may cause pain for the patient.

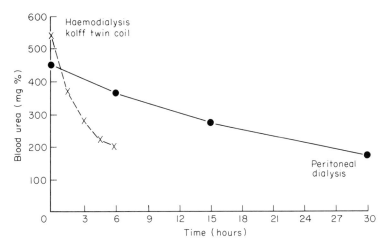

Fig. 10.1. Curve of blood urea levels after treatment of uraemia by peritoneal dialysis and haemodialysis.

Therefore peritoneal dialysis alone will not always suffice. Daily haemodialysis is more easily provided nowadays because nurses are well practised in its routine. Sophisticated monitoring both of the machine and of the patient's circulation makes it safer. Dialyser performance is more predictable. Access to the circulation can be achieved quickly using the Seldinger method to insert short Teflon catheters into the femoral veins, and once the first haemodialysis has been performed, a teflon silastic shunt can be electively sited in the forearm or at the ankle. The renal physician collaborating in the care of postoperative cardiac cases will be limited if he does not have both peritoneal dialysis and haemodialysis together with ultrafiltration techniques available.

(e) THE TECHNIQUE OF PERITONEAL DIALYSIS

The peritoneum has an area of approximately two square metres, and allows the exchange of electrolytes and urea and the loss of some protein. The tonicity of the dialysate can be varied by changing the concentration of dextrose, which controls the fluid exchange across the peritoneum. The absorbed dextrose can then be utilized and so acts as a protein sparer. A solution containing 1.36 g% of dextrose is used when there is no need to remove fluid from the patient, changing to a higher concentration to remove fluid when the patient is in cardiac failure with pulmonary or systemic oedema. The concentration of electrolytes of two commercially available solutions are shown in Table 10.2 and alternations of these produce any desired dextrose concentrations. Removal of water from the extracellular space is best carried out by alternating 1.36 and 6.36 g% dextrose solutions. The osmolality of the dialysis fluid is brought up to 330 mos nol/l.

Table 10.2. Solutions for peritoneal dialysis

	'Dialaflex 61'	*'Dialaflex 62'*
	g/l	g/l
Dextrose BP	13.6	63.6
Sodium Lactate BPC 1923	5.0	5.0
Sodium Chloride BP	5.6	5.6
Calcium Chloride BP	0.39	0.39
Magnesium Chloride Hexahydrate BPC 1934	0.15	0.15
Sodium Metabisulphite (Antioxidant)	0.05	0.12
	mmol/l	mmol/l
Sodium	140.4	140.4
Calcium	3.6	3.6
Magnesium	1.5	1.5
Total chloride	100.8	100.8
Lactate	44.6	44.6
Dextrose	13.6 (g/l)	63.6 (g/l)

Lactate from the dialysate is also absorbed and metabolised to bicarbonate in the liver. Urea, potassium, sulphate, phosphate, citrate, magnesium and calcium can be removed, and their clearance varies with the concentrations of the substance in blood and dialysis solution, the volume of the solution and the time that it is left in the peritoneal cavity (Fig. 10.2).

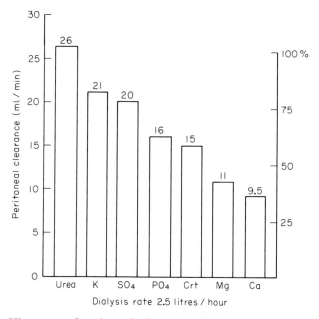

Fig. 10.2. Histogram of peritoneal clearance of potassium, sulphate phosphate, creatinine, magnesium and calcium at a peritoneal dialysis rate of 2.5 litres per hour.

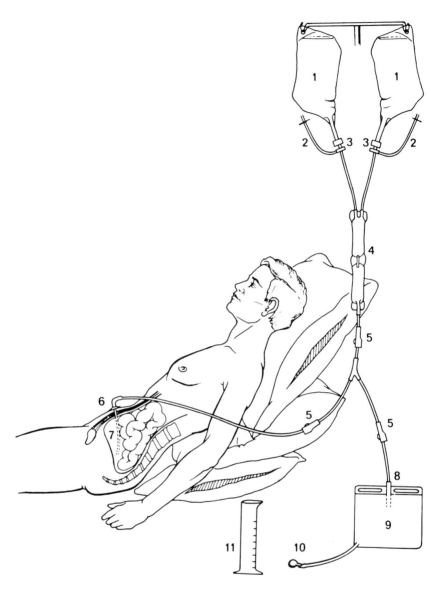

Fig. 10.3. Peritoneal dialysis. (1) 1-litre plastic bags containing dialysis solution. (2) Air vent with cotton wool air filter (does not work when wet); not needed with collapsible plastic bags. (3) 'Spike' contains fluid outlet and airway: non-return valve on airway. (4) Drip chamber. (5) Flow control. (6) Sterile dressing and adhesive plaster at insertion site. (7) Catheter lying in pelvis. (8) Non-return valve. (9) Sterile drainage bag. (10) Clamped drainage tube for emptying bag. (11) Graduated measuring cylinder. Reproduced from *The Renal Unit* by A. J. Wing and Mary Magowan with permission of the authors and MacMillan Press Ltd.

The peritoneal catheter and its metal stylet are inserted under local anaesthesia through the abdominal wall midway between the umbilicus and pubis, with the patient supine and the bladder empty. The special catheter is inserted deep into the pelvis, if necessary with the aid of fluid injections. The catheter is made of nylon, is slightly curved and has 80 tiny holes over the distal three inches to prevent omental plugging.

The catheter is connected to a Y drip set. One litre of pre-warmed dialysis fluid is run in as fast as possible and syphoned out immediately. After three

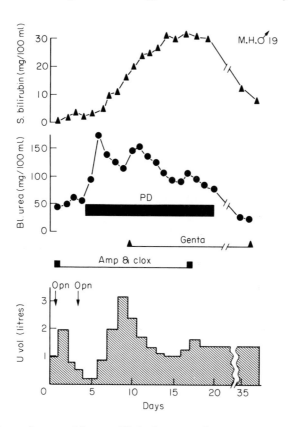

Fig. 10.4. Illustrative case history. Clinical course of acute renal failure following cardiac surgery in a 19-year-old man. A modified Fontan operation was carried out for single ventricle and pulmonary stenosis. Three days later a second operation was done as an emergency in order to repair the plication of the tricuspid valve. A period of hypotension followed this second operation and ATN supervened. Despite prompt return of urine output, peritoneal dialysis was required for 17 days until renal function recovered. Other problems in this patient were: septicaemia necessitating treatment with gentamicin (with blood level monitoring), ventilatory failure requiring tracheostomy, and hepatic failure with jaundice and a coagulation defect. Intravenous feeding was continued throughout this severe illness. (PD = peritoneal dialysis, amp. & clox = ampicillin and cloxacillin, genta = gentamicin, U = urine)

non-stop cycles to establish that the system is working well, a 'dwell time', when all taps are closed, is arranged so that a 1 litre cycle is completed every half hour and so that the times taken for run in and run out are as brief as possible. The closed system makes infection less likely (Fig. 10.3).

After cardiac surgery small volumes are better than large because the diaphragm may be pushed up by large volumes and embarrass cardiac and respiratory function. Additions to the units of dialysis fluid are heparin (100 mg) in the first few cycles to prevent fibrin plugs, and potassium (4 mmol/l) if the plasma potassium is normal. Culture of the fluid for organisms is performed each day.

The cycle is repeated half-hourly and will probably be required continuously for several days. Relatively normal chemistry is then maintained by dialysis for 12 hours daily and the patient can be fed. Excessive fluid shifts are avoided by measurement of the fluid exchanges in and out and by weighing the patient. Careful measurement of the central venous pressure is essential during peritoneal dialysis if the cardiac output is low. Marked variations in ventricular filling pressures can occur if a central venous catheter is not inserted and regularly monitored. Fluctuations are corrected by altering the dextrose concentration of the perfusate, by transfusing blood, plasma or saline or by parenteral feeding.

The complications of peritoneal dialysis are seldom serious. Abdominal pain from overdistension is treated by reducing the volume of fluid introduced and altering the position of the catheter. A vasovagal attack with hypotension and bradycardia sometimes occurs and is treated with atropine. Bleeding, either uraemic or surgical, round the tube is treated by stopping the heparin addition in the fluid and, if necessary, transfusion. Perforation of the intestine is rare. Oedema of the abdominal wall may be due to a side hole of the tube being outside the peritoneum and requires replacement of the tube. Poor recovery of dialysis fluid from the peritoneum is corrected by flushing the catheter with saline, partially withdrawing it or replacing it in a new quadrant of the abdomen.

Management of renal failure following cardiac surgery is typified by an illustrative case history (Fig. 10.4).

REFERENCES

ABEL R.M., WICK J., BECK C.H., BUCKLEY M.J. & AUSTEN W.G. (1974). Renal dysfunction following open-heart operations. *Arch. Surg. (Chicago)* **108**, 175

BENNETT W.M., SINGER I. & COGGINS C.H. (1970) A practical guide to drug usage in adult patients with impaired renal function. *J. Amer. med. Ass.* **214**, 1468.

CANTAROVICH F., LOCATELLI A., FERNANDEZ J.C., PEREZ LOREDO J. & CHRISTHOT J. (1971) Frusemide in high doses in the treatment of acute renal failure. *Postgrad. Med. J. Suppl.* to Vol. **47**, 13.

CASALI R., SIMMONS R.L., NAJARIAN J.S., VON HARATIZSCH B., BUSELMEIER T.J. & KJELLSTRAND, C.M. (1975) Acute renal insufficiency complicating major cardiovascular surgery. *Ann. Surg.* **181**, 370.

FLORES J., DIBONA D., BECK C.H. & LEAF A. (1972) The role of cell swelling in ischemic renal damage and the protective effect of hypertonic solute. *J. clin. Invest.* **51**, 118.

FLYNN C.T. (ed.) (1974) *Acute Renal Failure.* MTP, Lancaster, England.

GRECO F. DEL (1975) The kidney in congestive heart failure. *Mod. Concepts cardiovasc. Dis.* **44**, 47.

GRISMER J.T., LEVY M.J., LILLEHEI R.C., INDEGLIA R. & LILLEHEI C.W. (1964) Renal function in acquired valvular heart disease and effects of extracorporeal circulation. *Surgery* **55**, 24.

HILBERMAN M., MYERS B.D., CARRIE B.J., DERBY G., JAMISON R.L. & STINSON E.B. (1979) Acute renal failure following cardiac surgery. *J. thorac. cardiovasc. Surg.* **77**, 880.

KERR D.N.S. (1979) Acute renal failure. In *Renal Disease* 4th edition, p. 437, eds. D. A. K. Black and N. F. Jones, Blackwell Scientific Publications, Oxford.

KUEHNEL E., & BENNETT W. (1976) Acute renal failure: discussions in patient management. Henry Kimpton, London.

LEE H.A. (1978) The nutritional management of renal diseases. In *Nutrition in the Clinical Management of Disease*, ed. J.W.T. Dickerson and H.A. Lee. Edward Arnold, London.

LUKE R.G., BRIGGS J.D., ALLISON M.E.M. & KENNEDY A.C. (1970) Factors determining response to mannitol in acute renal failure. *Amer. J. med. Sci.* **259**, 168.

MIELKE J.E., HUNT J.C., MAHER F.T. & KIRKLIN J.W. (1966) Renal performance during clinical cardiopulmonary bypass with and without hemodilution. *J. thorac. cardiovasc. Surg.* **51**, 229.

PORTER G.A., & STARR A. (1969) Management of postoperative renal failure following cardiovascular surgery. *Surgery* **65**, 390.

POWERS S.R. JR., BOBA A., HOSTNIK W. & STEIN A. (1964) Prevention of postoperative acute renal failure with mannitol in 100 cases. *Surgery* **55**, 15.

TILNEY N.L., BAILEY G.L. & MORGAN A.F. (1973) Sequential system failure after rupture of abdominal aortic aneurysms; an unsolved problem in postoperative care. *Ann. Surg.* **178**, 117.

YEH T.J., BROCKNEY E.L., HALL D.P. & ELLISON R.G. (1964) Renal complications of open-heart surgery: predisposing factors, prevention and management. *J. thorac. cardiovasc. Surg.* **47**, 79.

CHAPTER 11

Cerebral Damage

Cerebral disturbances after cardiac surgery, whether psychiatric or giving rise to neurological signs, are usually due to organic damage to the brain which may be slight or so severe that it causes coma and death. Clinically the effects may be apparent immediately after surgery or may be delayed in their onset for hours or days.

1. Aetiology

Embolism and cerebral ischaemia are the two main causes of brain damage after cardiac surgery but intracranial haemorrhage, hypothermia and metabolic disturbances can sometimes be implicated.

a. EMBOLISM

Embolism during and after cardiac surgery may be due to air, thrombus, fat, calcium, fibrin or antifoam. Air embolism is still probably the most common cause of cerebral damage after cardiac surgery, although its incidence has been markedly diminished since it has been appreciated how much care has to be taken to remove air trapped in the left heart after open heart surgery. The nitrogen content of air is absorbed slowly, which makes air more dangerous than oxygen or carbon-dioxide embolism, both of which may also occur during cardiopulmonary bypass if frothing occurs in an oxygenator or if cold blood comes in contact with warm tissues.

Cerebral thrombo-embolism arises from clot in the left atrium and appendage in mitral valve disease dislodged at the time of surgery, particularly after closed mitral valvotomy where the appendage is entered with the finger. Left ventricular aneurysms often contain clot. Thrombosis on left atrial suture lines and prosthetic valves is another source of postoperative thrombo-embolism.

Fat embolism is caused when the fat globules that lie in the pericardium after median sternotomy incisions or after trauma to mediastinal fat are sucked by coronary aspirators into the extracorporeal equipment. It has also been reported after cardiac massage.

Calcium may be dislodged during manipulations on calcified valves. Antifoam embolism is today rare, occurring when it is washed off by prolonged flow over bubble-oxygenator defoaming chambers. Fibrin embolism has become recognised as an important cause of diffuse brain damage, some oxygenators being more likely to form multiple microemboli than others. Occasionally prosthetic material—patches, stitches, etc.—may reach the brain as emboli.

b. CEREBRAL ISCHAEMIA AND ANOXIA

Cerebral blood flow is controlled mainly by the carbon dioxide tension and the pressure in the cerebral vessels. Total circulatory arrest causes cerebral damage after three minutes at normal body temperatures and eight minutes at 30°C. The degree of damage is aggravated by periods of poor circulation before and after the anoxic insult.

Cerebral ischaemia is also caused by a very low cardiac output, a low flow from a pump oxygenator, or a low arterial carbon dioxide tension, the last of which occurs if pure oxygen is used in the oxygenator during cardiopulmonary bypass or if hyperventilation occurs during or after surgery. Marked desaturation of the arterial blood causes anoxia of the cerebrum and follows large right to left shunts, faulty oxygenation by the anaesthetist or pump oxygenator during surgery or pulmonary complications and ventilatory inadequacies afterwards.

c. INTRACRANIAL HAEMORRHAGE

Intracranial haemorrhage is not uncommon after cardiac surgery associated with bleeding diatheses or excessive anticoagulation. Subdural haematomata occur after cerebral dehydration with hypertonic solutions or, in infants, with the increased osmolarity of excessive electrolyte infusion. Berry aneurysms may rupture during hypertensive crises, particularly after coarctation surgery, and cause subarachnoid haemorrhage. A sustained rise of cerebral venous pressure from superior vena caval obstruction may cause petechial or subdural haemorrhages as well as cerebral oedema. Venous cross communications cannot be relied on to relieve a high intracerebral pressure if one jugular vein is obstructed.

d. OTHER CAUSES OF NEUROLOGICAL DISTURBANCES

Profound hypothermia of 15°C has been said to cause cerebral damage but the damage is more likely to be ischaemic than due to direct damage from the temperature.

Cerebral symptoms due to metabolic disturbances are rare, but neurological changes are seen in hypoglycaemia, diabetic coma, gross electrolyte imbalance or a very low pH.

Drugs, such as penicillin or lignocaine, may cause fits if given in excessive dosage, particularly if the former is added to the pump oxygenator prime.

e. PSYCHIATRIC DISTURBANCES

Psychiatric disturbances of various degrees from slight disorientation to major psychoses occur frequently after cardiac surgery. They are usually organic in origin associated with any of the causes of diffuse cerebral damage listed above, although a low cardiac output is probably the most common cause. The intensive therapy unit is also a cause of psychiatric disturbance, due to lack of sleep, fear of impending death and the general atmosphere of unreality.

2. Pathology

The pathology of cerebral damage varies according to its aetiology. The changes typical of ischaemia and anoxia consist of diffuse neuronal loss in the cerebral cortex, the medulla being less affected and sometimes allowing survival of a decerebrate patient. Cerebral oedema may or may not occur.

Clot and calcium embolism cause typical infarcts. Diffuse focal areas of cerebral damage have been described in many patients after open heart surgery and may be due to fibrin or air embolism.

3. Diagnosis

Clinically cerebral damage presents with neurological or psychiatric disturbances which may be obvious immediately after discontinuation of anaesthesia or be delayed in their onset for hours or days.

a. ASSESSMENT OF CEREBRAL DAMAGE

The possibility of delayed development of cerebral symptoms means that regular neurological examinations are necessary in the early days after cardiac surgery. In order to establish a baseline, a check of the patient's neurological state is carried out immediately after his return to the intensive care unit. The level of consciousness and the reaction and equality of the pupils are noted. Spontaneous movement of all four limbs is looked for. Response to commands is elicited, failing which muscle tone and reflexes are assessed. If any abnormal neurological signs are found, as full a neurological examination as possible is performed—basically the level of consciousness, pupil responses, muscle tone and reflexes.

A check on the neurological state is repeated regularly, the frequency depending on the state of the patient, but assessment at least once a day is necessary if pareses are not to be missed.

The active assistance of a neurologist is invaluable and he should be considered an essential part of the therepeutic team after cerebral damage has occurred.

b. NEUROLOGICAL DAMAGE

The clinical picture is related to the severity, site and nature of the cerebral lesion. The common neurological signs include various disorders of consciousness, unequal pupils, hemiparesis, convulsions, hyperpyrexia, hyperreflexia and extensor plantar responses. An electroencephalogram is of value in diagnosing and assessing brain damage, but needs expert interpretation. Lumbar puncture is rarely helpful.

Cerebral oedema is best diagnosed from expert neurological analysis of the changing signs, particularly of pupil enlargement, slowing pulse or spreading hemiparesis or hemi-sensory loss. Papilloedema on examination of the fundi suggests cerebral oedema but its absence does not exclude the diagnosis.

The CT scanner (coaxial tomography) has improved the accuracy of diagnosis of post operative cerebral damage. Cerebral infarction, haemorrhage, oedema, brain shift and subdural haematoma can readily be recognised. An isodense subdural haematoma may be missed by a CT scan but, if suspected, the total absence of cortical sulci and ventricles of smaller size than normal are indicative of its presence.

It is useful from the point of view of management and prognosis to classify patients loosely into three clinical groups.

Group I have slight cerebral damage. There is no loss of consciousness but drowsiness, irritability or mental confusion is present. The pupils are normal sized, equal and react to light. Neurological signs, such as hemiparesis or hemiplegia, are transient and recovery is rapid and complete.

Group II have moderate damage. The patient is usually semi-conscious or unconscious, with or without focal signs, and local and generalised twitchings and convulsions are common. The pupils may be unequal but they react to light. The limbs may be hypertonic or flaccid and the reflexes are variable in their responses. Recovery is slow but steady, although at times the condition remains static for a number of days and then again starts to improve.

Group III have severe damage. The patient is deeply unconscious with fixed and dilated pupils. The limbs are flaccid. The condition is irreversible and nearly always leads to death from respiratory and circulatory failure, although some patients survive with gross neurological defects. If the patients are artificially ventilated they may live for days or weeks. The electroencephalogram is helpful in determining irreversible cerebral damage if taken within the first two days. A flat trace virtually precludes recovery.

It must be pointed out that this is a rough grouping not based on any definite criteria and is useful only as an aid in the management of the patients. Some may not fall distinctly into a single group, while others may pass from one to another in the course of their illness.

c. PSYCHIATRIC DISTURBANCES

Psychiatric disturbances tend to be delayed until about the third to fifth postoperative day but may begin immediately and last days or weeks. Sleep deprivation and anxiety are common. Psychiatric disturbance varies from minor degrees of disorientation to severe psychoses of all types provoked by the mental stress of operations on 'the heart', but the most common abnormalities are confusional states and hallucinations.

Confusional states tend to occur when the cardiac output is low. The patient suffers from illusions with misinterpretation of sensory stimuli; disorientation in respect to himself, others, time and place; clouding of his consciousness so that he is only half awake; and fragmentation of speech and thought so that he uses wrong words and gives wrong answers to simple questions.

Hallucinations tend to occur when the cardiac output is once again improving.

4. Prevention of Cerebral Damage

Once the brain has been damaged, treatment has relatively little influence on the lesion so that prevention of cerebral damage is vital. An E.E.G. monitor in the operating theatres is invaluable in diagnosing poor cerebral perfusion and accelerating preventive measures.

Embolic damage is avoided during surgery by meticulous care in evacuating all air from the left heart and leaving a bleeding point in the ascending aorta as the circulation is being re-established after open heart surgery, removing all clot from the left atrium and appendage, arresting the heart before mobilizing ventricular aneurysms, avoiding as far as possible using blood spilt into the pericardium, washing the pericardium clear of fat before bypass begins, taking care not to allow calcium to fall into the cardiac chambers, filtering all blood sucked out of the heart before returning it to the oxygenator, and inserting special filters into the arterial return to remove microemboli of fibrin and red cell aggregates. After surgery the incidence of embolism is minimised by effective anticoagulation of patients who have had extensive left heart procedures or prosthetic valve replacements.

Ischaemic and anoxic cerebral damage is prevented by keeping the cardiac output adequate at all times, by efficient massage and pulmonary ventilation during cardiac arrest, by avoidance of a low CO_2 tension from hyperventilation during anaesthesia or in the intensive care unit, by keeping flow rates and carbon dioxide tensions during cardiopulmonary bypass normal and by proper care of the lungs after surgery.

Intracranial haemorrhage is avoided by reducing systemic hypertension if it occurs, avoiding superior vena caval obstruction, keeping anticoagulation under control after surgery, and using hypertonic solutions with care, particularly in infants when the osmolarity of the extracellular fluids can rise markedly.

Psychiatric disturbances can be largely prevented by careful preparation of the patient for the ordeal ahead with explanation of postoperative procedures. The intensive therapy unit manoeuvres can be modified to allow the maximum amount of sleep, isolating the patient as far as possible from emergency procedures or deaths of other patients, keeping to a minimum the number and noise of rhythmic signalling monitors, removing wires and tubes from the patient as soon as possible and providing radio, television, a clock and an outside window. Constant reassurance by nurses and doctors and avoidance of discussion of a conscious patient's condition round his bed help to prevent mental strain. Transfer of the patient from intensive therapy unit to a normal ward may be accompanied by a lack of security sometimes and reassurance is again needed. Regular visiting by relatives is also helpful.

5. Treatment of Cerebral Damage

The treatment of cerebral damage once it has occurred is not entirely satisfactory because few measures carry any degree of success and because neurological opinion differs on their efficacy.

The management of a patient suffering from brain damage depends upon the nature and severity of the injury and the associated neurological signs. If the patient is in cardiac or respiratory failure also, these are intensively treated because a persistent poor output of desaturated blood aggravates the original cerebral lesion. No measures to treat brain damage are undertaken that might adversely affect the cardiovascular and respiratory systems until the latter are in a satisfactory state. If the patient is being artificially ventilated, the $P\text{CO}_2$ is maintained near 30 mm Hg.

The management of cerebral damage may be considered in two parts: treatment of the brain damage itself and the prevention and treatment of its effects on the other systems. The aim is to preserve the rest of the body in as normal a physiological state as possible until the brain recovers. Available measures include drugs, dehydration and the use of steroids, hypothermia and hyperventilation.

a. DRUGS

Drugs such as sedatives, narcotics, anticonvulsants and tranquillisers are used to depress the activity of the nervous system in order to control restlessness, twitchings and convulsions because the cardiorespiratory state of these patients is often delicately balanced and any strain may lead to rapid deterioration. The drugs should be chosen and used with great care, taking into account their potential myocardial depressant effects. Papaveretum (Omnopon) (5–10 mg 4–6 hourly), phenobarbitone sodium (60–120 mg tds), paraldehyde (2–7 ml intramuscularly up to 50–60 ml in 24 hours) and phenytoin sodium (Epanutin 50 mg 6-hourly), given singly or together, have been found to be effective.

Even these at times fail to control involuntary movements and the use of muscle relaxants may be necessary. Muscle relaxants, such as curare and pancuronium, are valuable drugs in the management of patients with convulsions, as they have little depressant action on the circulation in the quantities used. An endotracheal tube is passed or tracheostomy performed, artificial ventilation is begun and curare or pancuronium given intravenously or intramuscularly as often as necessary to cause paralysis of all muscles. It is continued until restlessness and involuntary movements disappear and signs of recovery occur. If the patient is conscious although paralysed, sedatives such as omnopon or phenobarbitone are given in addition. Skilled nursing care is necessary in the management of these patients but any hazards associated with this form of therapy are outweighed by its benefits.

Psychiatric disturbances respond to chlorpromazine (25 mg i.m. every 4 hours) or tranquillizers such as diazepam (Valium). Occasionally major psychotic disturbances have to be treated with electro-convulsive therapy.

b. DEHYDRATION AND HYPOTHERMIA

Cerebral oedema may complicate anoxic brain damage, but there is no evidence that it plays an important part in diffuse embolic damage. Cerebral oedema causes an increase in brain volume and a rise in intracranial pressure which leads to further neuronal damage, obstruction of the circulation of the cerebrospinal fluid and interference with the blood flow in the cerebral vessels. Treatment is aimed at reducing the size of the brain and preventing the harmful effects of cerebral oedema, and may be achieved by the intravenous use of hypertonic solutions, hypothermia or steroids.

The effect of hypertonic solutions is only temporary but may be used if papilloedema is present. A 25% solution of mannitol may be given intravenously 3–4 hourly, fluid intake is limited and a careful check is kept on venous pressures, fluid balance, blood and urinary electrolytes and the haematocrit (PCV). Unless the patient shows signs of a quick recovery, it should be discontinued, because the use of hypertonic solutions can be succeeded by 'rebound' swelling. The use of hypertonic solutions is contraindicated when there is oliguria due to impaired renal function and used with care in the presence of a high left atrial pressure because they may lead to overloading of the circulation.

Moderate hypothermia, lowering the body temperature to about 33°C, has been used to protect the brain from the effects of various insults. Hypothermia reduces brain bulk when cerebral oedema is present, reduces the metabolic needs of the brain cells after anoxia or injury and may help to control the hyperpyrexia that follows certain types of brain damage. As the process of inducing hypothermia produces vasoconstriction, may cause dysrhythmias or lower the cardiac output, it should be used with great caution, if at all, in patients who are also suffering from cardiovascular insufficiency, which limits its use in cardiac surgery.

c. STEROID THERAPY

Probably the best therapeutic measure today is the use of steroids to control cerebral oedema and local reaction to the injury as far as possible. A steroid such as Dexamethasone is given as a 10 mg dose initially followed by 4 mg 6 hourly, tailing the dose off slowly after recovery has occurred. Steroids should be begun as soon as possible after the damage is incurred if they are to be maximally effective.

d. PREVENTION AND TREATMENT OF DETERIORATION OF OTHER SYSTEMS

Skilled nursing care is essential in the management of an unconscious patient. The patient's position is changed frequently and meticulous care is taken of the skin, eyes and mouth. Physiotherapy is carried out for the chest and limbs. A nasogastric tube is passed and the stomach emptied frequently, however mild the neurological signs, because accumulation of excessive gastric contents are not uncommon in the first few days and the consequences of aspirating stomach contents into the lungs are disastrous. Later the same tube can be used for feeding. A catheter is passed into the bladder and left in position. The fluid, electrolyte and the acid-base state are regularly checked and adequately controlled. The requisite amount of calories and vitamins are supplied.

Positive pressure ventilation is used by many units in the management of cerebral damage, initially with an endotracheal tube and, later if recovery is likely to be prolonged, via a tracheostomy. This ensures clearing of secretions and maintenance of full oxygenation of the blood. The P_{CO_2} is kept around 30 mmHg, though some units reduce it electively by hyperventilation to 20 mmHg, on the basis that metabolic acidosis in the damaged parts of the brain can be counteracted by a respiratory alkalosis and that the reduction of cerebral blood flow due to the low P_{CO_2} does not affect the vessels of the damaged area which are dilated and unresponsive.

e. MODIFICATION OF TREATMENT FOR VARYING DEGREES OF CEREBRAL DAMAGE

Having considered the available measures for treatment of cerebral damage, it remains to discuss how individual cases are managed.

Patients in Group I (mild neurological damage) require no treatment for the brain damage beyond drugs such as sedatives or narcotics but they are watched carefully until recovery is complete to prevent blood gas or circulatory inadequacy which may cause further cerebral damage. They need an intragastric tube and, sometimes, a urinary catheter if a full bladder is causing discomfort and restlessness. Psychiatric disturbances respond to tranquillizers and the passage of time—sometimes six months or more—but rarely electroconvulsive therapy is necessary. A surgeon or cardiologist who is not sufficiently specific about postoperative activity and an overprotective family may inhibit full recovery.

Patients in Group II (moderate neurological damage) are observed for a short while to assess their progress. If there are definite, rapid and continuing signs of recovery, they are managed as in Group I. If the condition remains static, or deteriorates, active treatment is started promptly. If cerebral oedema is present, dehydration therapy is begun with mannitol, and steroids given. In other cases, steroids alone are used. Hypothermia is used for hyperpyrexia, without reducing the temperature below normal if the cardiac state is unstable. If restlessness or convulsions are present, sedatives and anticonvulsants are given. An endotracheal tube is passed or tracheostomy performed if sputum retention is a problem, but the patient is artificially ventilated only if there is respiratory or cardiovascular insufficiency or if the patient needs to be paralysed for intractible convulsions and restlessness. The full regime for the management of an unconscious patient is then carried out. Most patients in this group will make a good recovery, though the time taken to improve varies from a few hours to two to three weeks.

Patients in Group III (severe neurological damage) are treated intensively along the lines of Group II, but the prognosis is poor and if they survive they are often left with neurological deficits. A flat EEG indicates irrecoverable damage and raises the question of discontinuation of treatment.

REFERENCES

AGUILAR M.J., GERBODE F. & HILL J.D. (1971) Neuropathological complications of cardiac surgery. *J. thorac. cardiovasc. Surg.* **61**, 676.

ASHMORE P.C., SVITEK V. & AMBROSE P. (1968) The incidence and effects of particulate aggregation and microembolism in pump oxygenator systems. *J. thorac. cardiovasc. Surg.* **55**, 691.

BLACHLY P.H. & BLACHLY B.J. (1968) Vocational and emotional status of 263 patients after heart surgery. *Circulation* **38**, 524.

BRIERLEY J.B. (1967) Brain damage complicating open heart surgery: a neuropathological study of 46 patients. *Proc. roy. Soc. Med.* **60**, 858.

BRIERLEY J.B., ADAMS J.H., GRAHAM D.I. & SIMPSON J.A. (1971) Neocortical death after cardiac arrest. *Lancet* **ii**, 560.

COHEN S.I. (1964) Neurological and psychiatric aspects of open heart surgery. *Thorax* **19**, 575.

CURRIE T.T., HAYWARD N.J., WESTLAKE G. & WILLIAMS J. (1971) Epilepsy in cardiopulmonary bypass patients receiving large intravenous doses of penicillin. *J. thorac. cardiovasc. Surg.* **62**, 1.

FRANK K.A., HELLER S.S., KORNFELD D.S. & MALM J.R. (1972) Longterm effects of open heart surgery on intellectual functioning. *J. thorac. cardiovasc. Surg.* **64**, 811.

GILBERSTADT H. & SAKO Y. (1967) Intellectual and personality changes following open heart surgery. *Arch. Gen. Psychiat.* **16**, 210.

GILMAN S. (1965) Cerebral disorders after open heart operations. *New England J. Med.* **272**, 489.

HARLEY H.R.S. (1964) The use of hypothermia and dehydration in the treatment of severe cerebral hypoxia. *Brit. J. Anaesth.* **36**, 587.

HAZAN S.J. (1966) Psychiatric complications following cardiac surgery. *J. thorac. cardiovasc. Surg.* **51**, 307.

HILL J.D., AGUILAR M.J., BARANCO A. DE LANEROLLE P. & GERBODE F. (1969) Neuropathological manifestations of cardiac surgery. *Ann. thorac. Surg.* **7**, 409.

JAVID H., TUFO H.M., NAJAFI H., DYE W.S., HUNTER J.A. & JULIAN O.C. (1969) Neurological abnormalities following open heart surgery. *J. thorac. cardiovasc. Surg.* **58**, 502.

KORNFELD D.S., ZIMBERG S. & MALM J.R. (1965) Psychiatric complications of open heart surgery. *New England J. Med.* **273**, 287.

ORR W.C. & STAHL M.L. (1977) Sleep disturbances after open heart surgery. *Amer. J. Cardiol.* **39**, 196.

TUFO H.M., OSTFIELD A.M. & SHEKELLE R. (1970) Central nervous system dysfunction following open heart surgery. *J. Amer. med. Ass.* **212**, 1333.

SUMMERS W.K. (1979) Psychiatric sequelae to cardiotomy. *J. cardiovasc. Surg.* **20**, 471.

WITOSZKA M.W., TAMURA H., INDEGLIA R., HOPKINS R.W. & SIMEONE F.A. (1973) Electroencephalographic changes and cerebral complications in open heart surgery. *J. thorac. cardiovasc. Surg.* **66**, 855.

CHAPTER 12

Hepatic Failure

Depression of hepatic function is a relatively rare complication of congenital cardiac surgery but is not uncommon after any prolonged period of low cardiac output and after surgery for acquired heart disease, particularly if more than one valve is affected. Damage to the liver at the time of surgery is aggravated by previous liver disease. Viral infections are the cause of hepatic failure occurring later in the convalescent period.

1. Aetiology

Jaundice may develop after cardiac surgery for a variety of causes. An increased pigment load follows blood transfusion and this is exaggerated by extravasated blood in the tissues. Older patients with pulmonary hypertension, tricuspid regurgitation and myocardial insufficiency are particularly likely to develop hepatic failure as a complication of cardiac surgery as it is in these patients that hepatic function may be depressed before and during surgery. Anaesthesia, particularly with halothane, hypothermia, a low flow with poor tissue perfusion from the pump oxygenator and a raised plasma haemoglobin aggravate these effects. The kidneys simultaneously suffer from reduced renal blood flow and renal failure may be associated with the hepatic damage.

In the postoperative period, a low cardiac output and tricuspid regurgitation with a high venous pressure may aggravate hepatic damage. The increasing application of tricuspid valvoplasty at the time of left heart surgery has markedly reduced the incidence and effects of the latter. Reduced portal venous flow is probably also important. Some drugs can cause jaundice, e.g. phenothiazines, anabolic steroids, many psychiatric drugs, sulphonamides, erythromycin, estolate, anti-tuberculous drugs and phenindione. Sepsis also produces jaundice.

Transfusion viral hepatitis may occur after cardiac surgery after an incubation period of 14–100 days or possibly more, after transfusion of blood containing any of at least three human viruses, namely A and B (previously termed infective and serum hepatitis), and an unidentified 'non-A, non-B' virus. Cytomegalovirus hepatitis may also occur.

2. Diagnosis of Liver Damage

Jaundice of the skin and sclerae is usually obvious when the level of bilirubin in the blood is above 3 mg% (50 μmol/l). Increasing jaundice and a rising blood bilirubin usually imply intrahepatic cholestasis of the bile canaliculi due to hepatic damage rather than to bile duct obstruction. Advanced signs of liver failure are a flapping tremor of the hands, bleeding from a reduced prothrombin level, and coma.

Other convenient tests of liver function that can be used after cardiac surgery are the alkaline phosphatase level (normally 3–13 KA units) and the prothrombin time. The serum glutamic and pyruvic oxaloacetic transaminases, aspartate and alanine amino-transferases are unreliable as alteration in their levels may accompany damage in other tissues. Australia antigen may be detected in the serum of patients with serum hepatitis before the onset of jaundice and even before the liver function tests become abnormal, and may persist for weeks afterwards.

3. Types of Jaundice

There are three clinical syndromes of jaundice that occur after cardiac surgery. The first arises early, within three days, and consists of jaundice, bilirubin in the urine and raised blood bilirubin and alkaline phosphatase levels but no other evidence of hepatic damage. It is essentially benign and resolves spontaneously within a week.

The second is a more serious type. It arises later, around the 5th to 7th day, in patients who have had a low cardiac output before or after surgery, is often associated with poor renal function and a rising blood urea, and tends to progress relentlessly to death from hepatic failure.

The third type occurs some two to three months after cardiac surgery, due to the patient having been infected with viral hepatitis from plasma or blood given at or after surgery.

Haemolysis from jet lesions of valve stenosis or regurgitation from prosthetic valves, etc. can cause a mild jaundice, but it is seldom marked enough to be confused with the other types from which it is distinguished by a blood bilirubin of less than 5 mg/100 ml (83 μmol/l) and which is unconjugated, a raised urinary urobilinogen and the absence of bilirubin in the urine.

4. Treatment

a. PREVENTION

Prevention of liver damage implies avoidance of a low cardiac output and tricuspid regurgitation at all times, which is not always possible. Tricuspid valvoplasty, by circumferential suture (De Vega) or Carpentier ring, if tricuspid regurgitation has been or is present at surgery is probably the most important single preventive measure. Drugs known to be associated with hepatic damage are avoided if the output is low. Blood for transfusion should be screened for Hepatitis B surface (Australia) antigen.

b. MANAGEMENT OF ESTABLISHED HEPATIC FAILURE

Treatment of established hepatic failure is disappointing, almost all patients dying of bleeding, renal failure or cardiac failure in two or three weeks.

Failure of drug detoxication in the liver makes patients sensitive to sedatives and analgesics, which should be avoided as far as possible. Diazepam (Valium) is used in small doses if possible, though the usual analgesics may have to be given if pain is marked.

Failure to synthesize blood coagulation factors is probably the most serious effect of hepatic damage after cardiac surgery. Fibrinogen, prothrombin, and factors V, VII, IX and X are involved. The prothrombin time is prolonged and patients tend to bleed from everywhere—the wounds, venepuncture sites, nose, bronchi, bowel, brain and pericardium. Thrombocytopenia and fibrinolysis may occur and aggravate the bleeding tendency. Treatment is extremely difficult and large quantities of fresh blood and fresh frozen plasma are necessary and have to be repeated often. Fluctuations of blood volume and atrial pressures aggravate any degree of cardiac failure and a central venous pressure line is essential while blood and plasma are being administered.

Ammonia is produced by bacterial action in the bowel and its accumulation can be reduced by limiting protein by mouth, giving the poorly absorbed oral antibiotic neomycin and by giving the laxative lactulose. Deranged carbohydrate metabolism may cause a low blood sugar which requires a periodic check. Glucose by mouth or intravenous infusion will be necessary to provide calorie intake and correct hypoglycaemia.

A general vasodilatation may be seen, associated with a good cardiac output, as the period of low cardiac output has often passed by the time that hepatic failure appears. The patient is pink and warm peripherally with dilated veins but the venous and arterial pressures fall. Treatment is disappointing, but transfusion of the appropriate fluid, depending on the haematocrit, has to be given to maintain an adequate ventricular filling pressure. Intravenous hydrocortisone has been tried but, although it may cause a temporary improvement, is seldom effective in the long term.

Uraemia and oliguria commonly accompany acute hepatic failure, sometimes due to coincident renal damage with acute tubular necrosis at the time of the original episode of low cardiac output but more often due to the typical renal disturbance that accompanies hepatic failure, when the tubules function satisfactorily but the renal plasma flow and glomerular filtration rate are reduced for reasons that are not known. Fluid retention tends to occur but the renal failure may be aggravated by diuretic therapy. The plasma sodium level may fall as sodium passes into the 'sick' cells. Peritoneal dialysis removes the water overload, lowers the blood urea and may remove some of the toxic products that accumulate from hepatic damage but seldom reverses the condition. A raised plasma potassium is unusual but, if present, it is lowered with glucose and insulin and ion exchange resins. Occasionally potassium supplements may be needed. Sodium is not given unless there is clear evidence of loss of sodium from the body.

The respiratory rate and depth increase due to stimulation of the respiratory centres, perhaps by ammonia. The Pco_2 falls and cerebral blood flow is reduced, accentuating the tendency to coma.

Failure of albumin synthesis causes a low serum albumin level and a tendency to fluid retention if the patient survives for more than three weeks, but few live this long when acute hepatic failure complicates cardiac surgery.

The final picture of hepatic failure is of a deeply jaundiced, over-breathing, vasodilated, hypotensive patient with a low venous pressure, comatose or nearly so, with respiratory and metabolic alkalosis, oliguric and uraemic and bleeding from one or more areas.

REFERENCES

BIRGENS H.S., HENDRICKSON J., MATZEN P. & POULSEN H. (1978) The shock liver: clinical and biochemical findings in patients with centrilobular liver necrosis following cardiogenic shock. *Acta Med. Scand.* **204**, 417.

LA MONT J.T. (1974) Postoperative jaundice. *Surg. Clin. N. America* **54**, 637.

LOCKEY E., MCINTYRE N., ROSS D.N., BROOKS E.S. & STURRIDGE M.F. (1967) Early jaundice after open heart surgery. *Thorax* **22**, 165.

MUNDTH E.D., KELLER A.R. & AUSTEN W.G. (1967) Progressive hepatic and renal failure associated with low cardiac output following open heart surgery. *J. thorac. cardiovasc. Surg.* **53**, 275.

NUNES G., BLAISDELL F.W. & MARGARETTEN W. (1970) Mechanism of hepatic dysfunction following shock and trauma. *Arch. Surg. (Chicago)* **11**, 546.

ROSSITER S.J., MILLER D.G., RANEY A.A., OYER P.E., REITZ B.A., STINSON E.B. & SHUMWAY N.E. (1979) Hepatitis risk in cardiac surgical patients receiving factor IX concentrates. *J. thorac. cardiovasc. Surg.* **78**, 203.

RUBINSON R.M., HOLLAND P., SCHMIDT P.J. & MORROW A.G. (1965) Serum hepatitis after open heart operations. *J. thorac. cardiovasc. Surg.* **50**, 575.

SALAM A.R.A., DRUMMOND G.B., BAULD H.W. & SCOTT D.B. (1976) Clearance of indocyanine green given as an index of liver function during cyclopropane anaesthesia and induced hypotension. *Brit. J. Anaesth.* **48**, 321.

SANDERSON R.G., ELLISON J.H., BENSON J.A. & STARR A. (1967) Jaundice following open heart surgery. *Ann. Surg.* **165**, 217.

THOMPSON D.S. & GRIEFENSTEIN F.E. (1974) Enzyme patterns reflecting response to anaesthesia and operation. *Southern Med. J.* **67**, 69.

CHAPTER 13

Haematological Disorders

Haematological disorders commonly met with in postoperative cardiac patients are anaemia, haemoconcentration, transfusion reactions and failure of haemostatic mechanisms.

1. Postoperative Anaemia

a. AETIOLOGY

Anaemia occurs frequently after cardiac surgery. Its causes include inadequate blood replacement, blood damage in extracorporeal circulation, haemolysis, infection, and the use of certain drugs.

A common cause of postoperative anaemia is inadequate replacement of blood lost from the intravascular compartment during and after surgery. Estimation of total blood loss may be inaccurate because blood lost from the intravascular compartment and lying in the tissues cannot be measured directly. In the postoperative period a variable quantity of blood remains inside the chest despite good drainage and a slight widening of the mediastinum on the chest radiograph may represent some 500 ml.

Blood damage in extracorporeal circulation is of a complex nature and causes accelerated destruction of red blood cells in the post-perfusion period. The haemoglobin commonly falls by 3 to 5 g%.

Intravascular haemolysis may be due to artificial valves, leaks around them or jets impinging on prosthetic material and may result in loss of iron through the kidneys. Some valves, particularly in their smaller sizes in the aortic area, are more prone to haemolysis than others. Beall disc and cloth covered Starr ball valves are examples. Subclinical haemolysis is usual in the presence of prosthetic valves and the serum haptoglobins are usually lowered but this does not require treatment. Tendencies to haemolysis, such as sickle cell syndromes, aggravate these effects.

Subacute bacterial endocarditis or protracted low grade infection is sometimes the cause of anaemia and, in susceptible individuals, certain drugs such as chloramphenicol, sulphonamides and acetazoleamide may result in bone marrow depression while others may cause haemolysis.

b. DIAGNOSIS

The haemoglobin and haematocrit levels are regularly checked in all patients. A low haemoglobin will aggravate the effects of other complications such as cardiac failure, and a level below 11 g% will cause symptoms such as tiredness, weakness, dyspnoea on slight exertion, or tachycardia. Unrecognised haemorrhage, e.g. from the bowel or retroperitoneally, is looked for in any patient with severe anaemia, particularly if he is on anticoagulants.

The precise diagnosis of the cause of anaemia in a complex postoperative haematological situation is difficult and can only be elucidated with the help of a haematologist and so is outside the scope of this book.

c. PREVENTION

Prevention of severe postoperative anaemia is by adequate blood replacement, avoidance of excessive damage to blood by extracorporeal apparatus, and preventing leaks around artificial valves.

d. TREATMENT

Severe anaemia (less than 9 g% haemoglobin) needs active treatment by blood transfusion. Packed cells are given in preference to whole blood to avoid overloading the circulation. 540 ml of ACD blood yields 260 ml of a packed red cell suspension and the following formula may help to estimate the amount required:

Mls of packed cell suspension required = 3.5 × haemoglobin × body weight in kilograms, where the haemoglobin is the difference between the desired and the actual levels of haemoglobin in grams per cent in the patient.

If iron deficiency is diagnosed from estimation of the serum iron, unsaturated iron binding capacity and, if necessary, bone marrow biopsy, iron should be given, but the diagnosis of iron deficiency is often difficult after cardiac surgery, in which case an arbitrary course of oral iron for a month is not unreasonable. Anaemia due to leaks around prosthetic valves or too small a ball valve in the aortic area causing haemolysis may respond to giving iron only or to blood transfusion but will require valve replacement if anaemia is marked.

2. Haemoconcentration

a. AETIOLOGY

The haemoglobin and haematocrit (packed cell volume) levels always reflect the same haematological abnormalities but in certain circumstances it is simpler to think of haematocrit rather than haemoglobin values. This applies particularly in problems of haemoconcentration. Normal haematocrit (PCV) values range from 36 to 49% in adults and from 25 to 38% in children, levels that are primarily dependent on the red cell concentration but are also affected by red cell size. When extracorporeal circulation with diluting fluids such as 5% dextrose or Ringer's lactate has been used, a low PCV immediately after cardiac surgery is due to haemodilution. It corrects itself within a short time and needs no treatment. A low value is also found in postoperative anaemia.

A raised PCV after cardiac surgery is seen normally in patients with cyanotic heart disease. When it occurs in others it is a sign of serious importance. Haemoconcentration reduces renal plasma flow, leads to an increase in viscosity of the blood and may cause 'sludging' of red cell aggregates in the microvasculature. The causes of a raised PCV in the postoperative period include a high preoperative level, a raised venous pressure, overtransfusion with blood and dehydration.

In patients with cyanotic heart disease, the PCV may be normal at the end of the operation because of haemodilution during the perfusion but starts to rise again as fluid leaves the intravascular department. A high systemic venous pressure above 12 mm Hg measured from the sternal angle will cause the fluid part of the blood to be driven out into the tissues. Such a high venous pressure may follow congestive cardiac failure or overtransfusion with blood. Changes in the osmolarity of the plasma proteins and in the permeability of the capillaries also may allow fluid loss. Dehydration is another cause of a raised PCV.

b. DIAGNOSIS AND TREATMENT

Diagnosis is made by the laboratory or with a microcentrifuge in the intensive care unit during the first few days. The PCV is repeated frequently in the immediate postoperative period as marked changes may occur within a few hours.

If the haematocrit level is above 45% and the ventricular filling pressure is too low, plasma or a plasma substitute such as albumin is used instead of blood. If the PCV is very high (e.g. above 55%) and no further plasma expansion is required for treatment of the cardiac condition, blood can be carefully withdrawn, watching the venous pressures, and replaced by plasma.

3. Complications of Blood Transfusion

The postoperative cardiac patient is exposed not only to the risks inherent in any blood transfusion but also to the hazards of rapid transfusion of large quantities of blood. Complications occur in some 2–5% of all transfusions and may be minor or so severe as to cause death.

a. TRANSFUSION REACTIONS

Transfusion of incompatible blood produces a haemolytic transfusion reaction which is due to an increased rate of disruption of red cells of the donor or recipient. Its early signs and symptoms are lumbar pain, shivering, faintness, fever, and sometimes circulatory collapse, all of which may however be masked by anaesthesia or heavy sedation. Jaundice, haemoglobinuria and acute renal failure may follow after a variable period. The diagnosis of a haemolytic reaction is established by examination of the blood and urine when the presence of haemoglobinaemia, methaemalbuminaemia or haemoglobinuria is direct proof of intravascular haemolysis. This, however, is complicated by the fact that after bypass most patients have signs of intravascular haemolysis.

Sometimes a haemorrhagic reaction is present in addition, due to liberation of a thromboplastinlike substance into the bloodstream from the haemolysed red cells, which leads to intravascular coagulation and excessive consumption of clotting factors—known variously as the defibrination syndrome, disseminated intravascular coagulation (DIC) or consumptive coagulopathy. Persistent bleeding from the chest accompanied by oozing from the whole surgical field, prolonged bleeding and coagulation times, fibrinogenopenia, hypoprothrombinaemia and thrombocytopenia are usually also present and there may be increased activity of the fibrinolytic system.

As soon as a reaction to incompatible blood is suspected, the transfusion is stopped. Blood samples (one clotted and one anticoagulated with heparin) are taken and all bottles from which blood has been transfused are kept and sent to the laboratory. If blood loss continues and needs to be replaced, fresh compatible blood is used. Cardiac failure is corrected in the usual manner. Making the urine alkaline is of doubtful value but hydrocortisone may be given. Acute renal failure often follows a haemolytic reaction and is treated as in Chapter 10.

b. OTHER REACTIONS

Febrile reactions after blood transfusion are due to the presence of pyrogens and last a short time (some 8 to 12 hours). Allergic reactions, such as urticaria and asthma, may follow an antibody/antigen reaction between the donors and recipients of blood. They are treated with antihistamine drugs.

High fever, rigors and circulatory collapse may follow transfusion of infected blood, which may have become contaminated at the time of collection, during storage or during the transfusion, particularly if other drugs have been injected into the blood transfusion bottle. Depending on the infecting organisms, the blood may or may not be haemolysed. Careful collection and storage will help to prevent contamination of blood but organisms may occasionally enter the blood and multiply during storage at

4°C. Also, if blood is allowed to remain at a high room temperature for some hours, it may become infected with rapidly multiplying organisms, for which reason blood which has been standing at room temperature for more than five hours is best discarded.

Treatment of infective reactions consists of taking blood cultures followed by treatment with wide spectrum antibiotics. Infective and serum hepatitis (A and B with 'non A and non B') are the most feared infective complications of blood transfusion. Donors are screened for Hepatitis B surface (Australia) antigen. Malaria and syphilis may also be transmitted by transfusion of fresh blood.

A syndrome of fever, splenomegaly and increased numbers of mononuclear cells in the blood has been entitled the 'post-perfusion syndrome' and 'atypical mononucleosis'. Its aetiology is not known for certain but is presumed to be due to a virus, possibly the cytomegalovirus. This is diagnosed by high titres against cytomegalovirus in the serum. Its course is usually benign and requires no special treatment.

4. Failure of the Haemostatic Mechanisms

Bleeding after cardiac surgery and extracorporeal circulation can be a major and complex problem. When the bleeding site is inaccessible, it is often difficult to determine how much of the bleeding is due to inadequate surgical haemostasis and how much to failure of the haemostatic mechanisms, whether or not blood tests demonstrate depletion of the haemostatic reserve, because coagulation defects aggravate surgical bleeding and blood replacement with old blood, necessarily deficient in clotting factors, aggravates coagulation defects.

a. AETIOLOGY

Disorders of the haemostatic mechanisms may be due to circulating heparin, haemostatic abnormalities and thrombocytopenia.

Circulating heparin, inadequately neutralised, is a common cause of bleeding after cardiac surgery. Recrudescence of heparin activity after it has been effectively neutralised also occurs, the so-called heparin rebound, the cause of which is unknown but which may be due to heparinized blood being returned to the circulation from stagnant peripheral vessels, or to fibrinolytic degradation of the heparinprotamine complex. Lengthening of the thrombin time when it has been previously returned to normal by protamine may also be due to diminished fibrinogen levels or circulating products of fibrinolytic digestion of fibrinogen, but the thrombin time nevertheless usually returns to normal on giving more protamine, suggesting that reappearance of heparin is the most common cause of this phenomenon. An excessive dose of protamine may also prolong the coagulation time but this rarely occurs.

Haemostatic abnormalities may be present in some patients before operation. In severely cyanotic heart disease deficiencies of clotting factors, evidence of intravascular coagulation, thrombocytopenia or fibrinolysis may be found. Any coincidental bleeding diathesis may also be present but this is usually apparent from the history if it is carefully taken.

Cardiopulmonary bypass may directly reduce clotting factors. Early stages of the clotting sequence are activated by circulation of blood through an oxygenator and contact of blood with foreign surfaces. Without adequate heparinization and if traumatic extracorporeal apparatus is used, intravascular coagulation may be initiated and various clotting factors reduced. In addition, dilution by priming solutions for heart/lung machines reduces the concentration of clotting factors in the plasma, which is of particular importance in polycythaemic patients who have a low plasma volume.

Thrombocytopenia is invariable after cardiopulmonary bypass, the platelet count falling to half or one-third of the preoperative level within the first few minutes of perfusion. In addition, there is a secondary drop in the platelet count on the second postoperative day, which may last for about a week. The remaining platelets are usually adequate for haemostasis provided intravascular coagulation does not occur. Rarely thrombotic thrombocytopenic purpura, a variant of the defibrination syndrome (DIC, page 169) may be seen causing patchy ischaemia of the skin, purpura, and a sharp drop in the platelet count to very low levels, e.g. 1000 per cu mm. Its cause is unknown though it is often associated with a persistently low cardiac output.

Increased fibrinolytic activity occurs during cardiopulmonary bypass and if excessive or prolonged, may lead to bleeding. There may be an increase in the plasminogen activator activity or free circulating plasmin may be present in the blood. It usually returns to normal within a few hours of the end of perfusion. Menstruation alters the clotting state of the patient by lowering the platelet level, increasing the red cell fragility and activating fibrinolysis. Authorities differ on the degree and exact timing of these changes which occur unpredictably in any given patient, but the day before and the first two days of menstruation form the peak.

b. PREVENTION

At the time of cardiopulmonary bypass, adequate doses of heparin, and subsequently of protamine, are given, trauma to the blood in the oxygenator and coronary suction apparatus is reduced to a minimum, and blood used to prime the heart/lung machine is as fresh as possible. Haemodilution with non-blood primes, if not carried to extremes, appears to reduce postoperative blood loss.

Surgical haemostasis is carried out meticulously before closing the chest because there is always some deficiency of coagulation after cardiopulmonary bypass or if coumarin derivatives have been given. The degree of haemostasis that is adequate for general thoracic surgery is not sufficient to prevent haemorrhage after long periods of cardiopulmonary bypass particularly if profound hypothermia has been used. If surgical haemorrhage occurs, coagulation defects associated with massive transfusions of stored blood are added to the previous deficiencies.

c. DIAGNOSIS AND MANAGEMENT

(i) GENERAL MEASURES

Recognition of those patients who are likely to bleed at the time of cardiac surgery may allow the introduction of special measures to prevent postoperative haemorrhage. The history is the critical investigation. A history of excessive bleeding after minor injury, or prolonged bleeding after tooth extraction or other trauma, suggests the necessity for screening tests, whereas a history of normal haemostasis after several previous surgical traumata virtually precludes a clinically significant coagulation defect. Patients already on anticoagulants or who are polycythaemic are also at risk.

The cause of postoperative bleeding, even in the presence of detectable defects of the coagulation mechanism, is often surgical in origin because bleeding vessels have been overlooked at surgery or have begun to bleed again afterwards. Stopping a single important bleeding point often causes an oozing wound to become dry.

Fresh blood, preferably transfused at once from a previously crossmatched donor, is the single most useful factor when a major haemostatic defect cannot be identified, and every effort is made to obtain suitable donors if patients continue to bleed or are being returned to the operating theatre for bleeding. Fresh or fresh-frozen plasma is also useful.

(ii) POSTOPERATIVE SCREENING TESTS OF THE HAEMOSTATIC MECHANISM

If bleeding is considerable after cardiac surgery, or a failure of the haemostatic mechanism is suspected, a standard series of screening tests will rapidly eliminate obvious abnormalities of coagulation and allow specific treatment to be instituted.

1. *Thrombin time and Arvin time*

Arvin (Ancrod) clots fibrinogen but is not inhibited by heparin. A normal Arvin time combined with a prolonged thrombin time suggests that fibrinogen is present and is clottable and that the prolonged thrombin time is probably due to circulating un-neutralised heparin. If there is the least prolongation of the thrombin time, a further dose of protamine is given, equivalent to a quarter of the initial protamine dose given at the end of cardiopulmonary bypass. Haematologists often advise that minimal prolongations of the thrombin time do not need correction. While this is true in general and if there are no other haemostatic abnormalities, dramatic improvement in bleeding after cardiopulmonary bypass is often seen when a small prolongation is corrected by administration of further protamine.

2. *Sharp's fibrinogen titre and thrombin time*

When circulating heparin has been fully neutralised, or has not been given, a Sharp's fibrinogen titre and thrombin time are performed. If the fibrinogen titre is normal and the thrombin time prolonged, adequate fibrinogen is present but breakdown products (FDPs) of fibrinogen are probably circulating, suggesting that some fibrinolysis has occurred. The test for FDPs should be done. Active fibrinolysis, likely to be clinically important, will be shown by dissolution of the clots in the Sharp's test. Even if fibrinolysis is marked in vitro, antifibrinolytic drugs are given only if active bleeding is occurring. Associated clotting deficiencies (fibrinogen, factor V or factor VIII) increase the significance of fibrinolysis.

Treatment consists of giving antifibrinolytic drugs, such as epsilon aminocaproic acid (Epsikapron: 4–5 g four-hourly) or tranexamic acid (Cyklokapron: 1 g eight hourly) till the bleeding stops. Unnecessary use of these drugs may result in clotted haematomas being retained in the pleura and pericardium.

If the fibrinogen titre is reduced, other clotting factors may have been consumed also. Fibrinogen may be estimated and other tests performed, which will depend on local haematological facilities.

3. *Fibrinogen estimation*

A markedly reduced level of fibrinogen (below 100 mg%) is corrected with intravenous fibrinogen concentrate. The amount to be given is calculated from the formula:

Total fibrinogen deficit = Fibrinogen deficit in g per 100 ml of plasma × body weight in kg × 0.41.

4. *Platelets*

A platelet count will show whether thrombocytopenia is severe enough to account for bleeding. Platelet counts below 5000 per cu mm are treated with transfusion of fresh blood, platelet-rich plasma or a platelet concentrate.

The low platelet count associated with thrombotic thrombocytopenic purpura is characterised by a rapid continued fall of platelets to very low levels (page 169). The treatment of this condition is at present (1981) controversial and depends on subtle combinations of heparin and antiplatelet drugs for which the advice of a haematologist is essential.

REFERENCES

ANDERSEN M.N., GABRIELI E. & ZIZZI J.A. (1965) Chronic hemolysis in patients with ball valve prostheses. *J. thorac. cardiovasc. Surg.* **50**, 501.

BELL R.E., PETUOGLU S. & FRASER R.S. (1967) Chronic haemolysis occurring in patients following cardiac surgery. *Brit. Heart J.* **29**, 327.

BENTALL H.H. & ALLWORK S.P. (1968) Fibrinolysis and bleeding in open-heart surgery. *Lancet* **i**, 4.

BOYD A.D., ENGELMAN R.M., BEAUDET R.L. & LACKNER H. (1972) Disseminated intravascular coagulation following extracorporeal circulation. *J. thorac. cardiovasc. Surg.* **64**, 685.

FRIEDENBERG W.R., MYERS W.D., PLOTKA E.D., BEATHARD J.N., KUMMER D.J., GATLIN P.F., STOIBER D.L., RAY J.F. & SAUTTER R.D. (1978) Platelet dysfunction associated with cardiopulmonary bypass. *Ann. thorac. Surg.* **25**, 298.

GADBOYS H.L. & LITWAK R.S. (1963) The postperfusion haematocrit. *J. thorac. cardiovasc. Surg.* **46**, 772.

GARCIA J.B., PAKRASHI B.C., MARY D.A., TANDON R.K. & IONESCU M.I. (1973) Postoperative blood loss after extracorporeal circulation for heart valve surgery. *J. thorac. cardiovasc. Surg.* **65**, 487.

GOMES M.M.R. & McGOON D.C. (1970) Bleeding patterns after open-heart surgery. *J. thorac. cardiovasc. Surg.* **60**, 87.

GRALNICK H.R. & FISCHER R.D. (1971) The hemostatic response to open-heart operations. *J. thorac. cardiovasc. Surg.* **61**, 909.

HARDAWAY R.M. (1967) Disseminated intravascular coagulation in experimental and clinical shock. *Amer. J. Cardiol.* **20**, 161.

HERR R., STARR A., McCORD C.W. & WOOD J.A. (1965) Special problems following valve replacement: Embolus, leak, infection and red cell damage. *Ann. thorac. Surg.* **1**, 403.

INDEGLIA R.A., SHEA M.A., VARCO R.L. & BERNSTEIN E.F. (1968) Erythrocyte destruction by prosthetic heart valves. Circulation Supp. 2, **37** and **38**, 86.

INGLIS, T.C.M., BREEZE G.R., STUART J., ABRAMS L.D., ROBERTS K.D. & SINGH S.P. (1975) Excess intravascular coagulation complicating low cardiac output. *J. Clin. Path.* **28**, 1.

INGRAM G.I.C. (1967) Current views on haemostasis. *Practitioner* **199**, 5.

KALTER R.D., SAUL C.M., WETSTEIN L., SORIANO C. & REISS R.F. (1979) Cardiopulmonary bypass: associated haemostatic abnormalities. *J. thorac. cardiovasc. Surg.* **77**, 427.

KAUL T.K., CROW M.J., RAJAH S.M. DEVERALL P.B. & WATSON D.A. (1979) Heparin administration during extracorporeal circulation: heparin rebound and postoperative bleeding. *J. thorac. cardiovasc. Surg.* **78**, 95.

DE LEVAL M.R., HILL J.D., MIELKE C.H., MACUR M.F. & GERBODE F. (1975) Blood platelets and extracorporeal circulation. *J. thorac. cardiovasc. Surg.* **69**, 144.

LEFEMINE A.A., MILLER M. & PINDER G.C. (1974) Chronic hemolysis produced by cloth-covered valves. *J. thorac. cardiovasc. Surg.* **67**, 857.

McKAY D.G. & MÜLLER-BERGHAUS G. (1967) Therapeutic implications of disseminated intravascular coagulation. *Amer. J. Cardiol.* **20**, 392.

MARGARETTEN W. (1967) Local tissue damage in disseminated intravascular clotting. *Amer. J. Cardiol.* **20**, 185.

PORTER J.M. & SILVER D. (1968) Alterations in fibrinolysis and coagulation associated with cardiopulmonary bypass. *J. thorac. cardiovasc. Surg.* **56**, 869.

RODGERS B.M. & SABISTON D.C. (1969) Hemolytic anaemia following prosthetic valve replacement. *Circulation Supp.* 1, **39** and **40**, 155.

ROTHNIE N.G. & KINMONTH J.B. (1960) Bleeding after perfusion for open heart surgery. *Brit. med. J.* **1**, 73.

RUBINSON R.M., MORROW A.G. & GEBEL P. (1966) Mechanical destruction of erythrocytes by incompetent aortic valvular prostheses. *Amer. Heart J.* **71**, 179.

SHARP A.A. (1977) Diagnosis and management of disseminated intravascular coagulation. *Brit. med. Bull.* **33**, 265.

TICE D.A., REED G.E., CLAUSS R.H. & WORTH M.H. (1963) Hemorrhage due to fibrinolysis occurring with open-heart operations. *J. thorac. cardiovasc. Surg.* **46**, 673.

UMLAS J. (1975) Fibrinolysis and disseminated intravascular coagulation in open heart surgery. *Transfusion* **16**, 460.

WAGSTAFFE J.G., CLARKE A.D. & JACKSON P.W. (1972) Reduction of blood loss by restoration of platelet levels using fresh autologous blood after cardiopulmonary bypass. *Thorax* **27**, 410.

WALLACE H.W. & BLAKEMORE W.S. (1970) Intravascular and extravascular hemolysis accompanying extracorporeal circulation. *Circulation* **42**, 521.

YACOUB M.H., KOTHARI M. KEELING D., PATTERSON M. & ROSS D.N. (1969) Red cell survival after homograft replacement of the aortic valve. *Thorax* **24**, 283.

CHAPTER 14

Cardiac Arrest

Cardiac arrest can be defined as the cessation of an effective circulation which may be due to cardiac asystole, ventricular fibrillation or a grossly inadequate cardiac output, the last being due to poor myocardial contractions or extreme tachycardia or bradycardia.

1. Aetiology

The causes of cardiac arrest include hypoxia and irritability of the myocardium, dysrhythmias, coronary artery obstruction, hypothermia, certain drugs and perhaps vasovagal reflexes.

Hypoxia of the myocardium may be caused by a low arterial oxygen saturation in the blood supplying the coronary arteries. This is less likely to cause cardiac arrest than occlusion of the vessels themselves, when differential oxygenation of neighbouring parts of the myocardium may produce an electrical potential that initiates ventricular fibrillation.

Hypothermia increases myocardial excitability, when ventricular fibrillation may occur spontaneously. Persistent hypothermia is not uncommon after operations involving cooling because of cooled muscle masses at the time of surgery which had not been fully rewarmed. Massive postoperative blood transfusion of cold blood in the treatment of haemorrhage can also produce hypothermia which, combined with the hypotension which may occur if blood replacement is inadequate, makes ventricular fibrillation a risk.

Drugs such as digitalis, quinidine and anaesthetic agents may cause ventricular fibrillation. A low serum potassium level, which may follow the diuresis of dilution perfusions, prolonged diuretic treatment, alkalosis or positive pressure ventilation, may potentiate the action of digitalis and produce ventricular tachycardia and fibrillation. A high serum potassium level causes weak myocardial contractions and ultimately cardiac arrest. Vasovagal reflexes may act similarly, the stimuli being inhalation of vomit, tracheostomy, tracheal intubation and suction, although the cardiac arrest is more probably anoxic in origin.

Postural hypotension, which can follow sitting up an already hypotensive

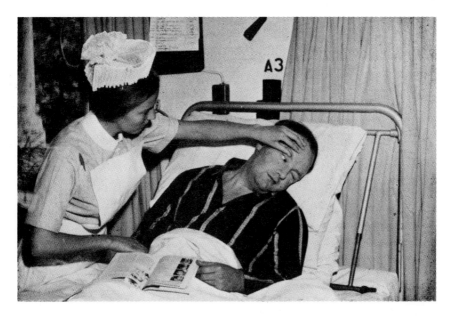

Fig. 14.1. The diagnosis of cardiac arrest is made on four signs: unconsciousness, apnoea, absent pulse and dilating pupils. These mean that the circulation is inadequate and treatment is started immediately.

patient for a radiograph, can also precipitate cardiac arrest. Arrhythmias such as ventricular tachycardia and complete heart block may be complicated by cardiac asystole or fibrillation.

Cardiac arrest usually has multiple causes, such as a combination of hypoxia, digitalis overdosage and a low serum potassium, or no obvious cause at all. The importance of trying to identify a cause is in order to correct it during and after resuscitation.

2. Diagnosis of Circulatory Arrest

Some sudden deterioration in the patient's condition commonly attracts attention (Fig. 14.1). He collapses, becomes unconscious, stops breathing and may twitch or convulse. The diagnosis is confirmed by finding that the pulse is absent. The pulse is best sought in a major vessel, either the carotid or femoral artery, but the radial artery is the most familiar to many and if a nurse is uncertain of her ability to find the larger vessels she should use the radial. The pupils start to dilate 30–45 seconds after cardiac arrest.

If the electrocardiogram is being monitored, the oscilloscope may show asystole (Fig. 14.2), ventricular fibrillation (Fig. 14.3), extreme bradycardia (Fig. 14.2) or tachycardia or relatively normal complexes. The ECG is never

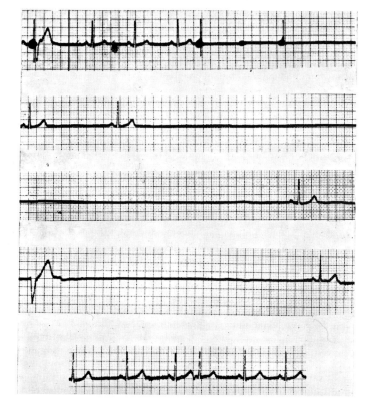

Fig. 14.2. Electrocardiogram of sinus bradycardia followed by cardiac asystole. Lowest line shows reversion to sinus rhythm.

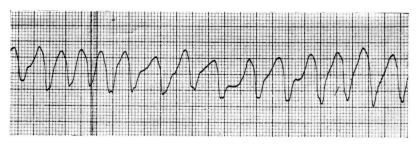

Fig. 14.3. Electrocardiogram of ventricular fibrillation.

used as the sole evidence of cardiac arrest because a common cause of a flat trace on the oscilloscope is a lead becoming detached from the patient.

The four signs—unconsciousness, apnoea, absent pulses and dilating pupils—mean circulatory arrest. No further time is wasted in refinements of diagnosis: the person making the diagnosis calls for help and starts treatment immediately.

3. Treatment of Cardiac Arrest

Resuscitation is started as soon as cardiac arrest is recognized, for two reasons. The brain will survive unharmed for only three minutes once its circulation ceases and the heart itself suffers from the absence of coronary blood flow, with the result that the longer resuscitation is postponed the less likely is restoration of a normal beat. Resuscitation is most often successful when the person making the diagnosis of arrest institutes the treatment.

Treatment is divided into three stages: provision of an artificial circulation of oxygenated blood, restoration of a normal beat, and after-care and treatment of complications.

a. PROVISION OF AN ARTIFICIAL CIRCULATION OF OXYGENATED BLOOD

The provision of an artificial circulation of oxygenated blood requires external cardiac massage and artificial ventilation. Both can be performed simultaneously if two people are present but if a nurse is alone she has to alternate between the two.

(i) EXTERNAL CARDIAC MASSAGE

The pillows are pulled out and the patient laid flat (Fig. 14.4). Most hospital beds are too high and too wide for efficient cardiac massage to be performed with the operator standing on the floor. It is best done with the operator kneeling on the bed. The costal margin is palpated and the lower half of the sternum identified. The heel of one hand is placed over the lower half of the sternum, and the other hand on top of the first. Keeping the arms straight, the sternum is quickly but firmly depressed $1\frac{1}{2}$ in to 2 in in an adult (less for children) 60–80 times a minute, allowing for pauses for artificial ventilation. This means in practice six depressions in 3 seconds, followed by a single inflation of the lungs by the anaesthetist lasting 2 seconds.

The heart is compressed between the sternum and vertebral column and its contained blood ejected into the pulmonary artery and aorta. Pressure is only applied over the lower half of the sternum because force applied elsewhere may fracture ribs or damage the liver or spleen. The chest is allowed to expand completely after each compression, or the venous return will be impeded and the cardiac ouput diminished. Venous return is also aided by raising the patient's legs.

External massage should be performed with the patient lying on a firm surface and intensive care unit beds should therefore have hard frames rather than springs. A fracture board or special cardiac massage board is inserted under the patient as soon as possible if he is in a spring bed, but this should not delay the start of cardiac massage and artificial respiration.

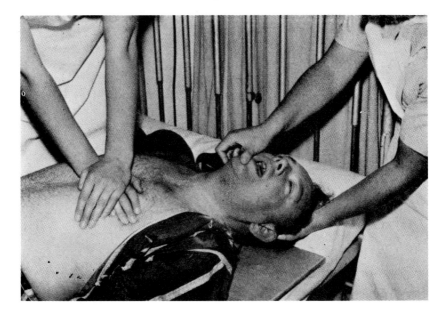

Fig. 14.4. The bedclothes are thrown back, pillows pushed out and the patient pulled flat. Kneeling on the bed, the nurse places her hands one over the other over the lower half of the sternum and starts external compression with a quick but firm compression. The airway is cleared by extending the head and neck with the left hand and pulling the jaw forward with the thumb of the right hand on the chin and the fingers behind the angle. Foreign material is removed.

(ii) ARTIFICIAL VENTILATION

In any method of artificial ventilation there are three basic essentials: the first is to clear and maintain the airway, the second is to get an airtight fit with the patient's face if a mask is used, and the third is to see that the chest actually expands during each inflation. The patient must be allowed to exhale completely between inflations.

Before any form of artificial ventilation is begun, the upper airway is cleared (Fig. 14.4). In an unconscious patient the tongue falls back against the posterior pharyngeal wall and the airway may be further obstructed by regurgitated material or an inhaled foreign body. The head and neck are extended and the jaw pulled forward. This is best achieved with the thumb on the chin and a finger behind the angle of the jaw which results in the tongue being lifted forward with the jaw. This tends to open the mouth and any foreign material can then be removed with a finger or sucker. The jaw must be kept forward throughout the period of artificial ventilation.

Ventilation can be performed with an Ambu bag and mask (Fig. 14.5), with a Brook or similar airway, or by mouth-to-mouth respiration (Fig. 14.6). Mouth-to-mouth ventilation can occasionally be life-saving but an Ambu

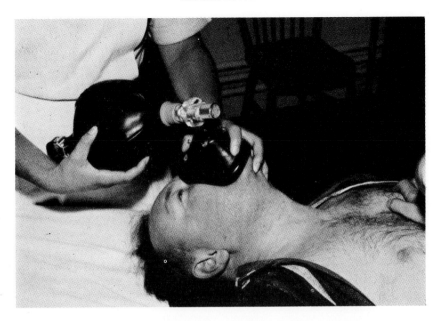

Fig. 14.5. The facemask of the Ambu bag is tightly applied, maintaining extension of the head. The bag is compressed between the nurse's hand and chest. No leak should be heard and the patient's chest must expand with each inflation.

bag or Brook airway is generally available in hospital. If the patient is already being ventilated with a tracheostomy or endotracheal tube, the ventilator is disconnected and hand inflation with an anaesthetic bag and 100% oxygen begun.

In practice it is difficult to perform ventilation while external cardiac massage is being performed and the person performing cardiac massage should pause every sixth compression to allow time for one good inflation. If a nurse is alone, massage is stopped every sixth compression while she quickly inflates the patient herself.

(iii) ASSESSMENT OF THE EFFECTIVENESS OF MASSAGE AND VENTILATION

Efficient external cardiac compression results in a pulse being felt in a major artery which is palpated by the person performing artificial ventilation. It is not easy sometimes to distinguish arterial from venous pulsation under these circumstances. The return of circulation to the brain results in the pupils shrinking to a normal size, and sometimes the patient will start to make respiratory efforts and regain consciousness. Adequate ventilation is assessed by expansion of the chest with each inflation, lessening of the cyanosis and an adequate partial pressure of oxygen on an arterial blood sample taken from an indwelling radial line or by femoral arterial puncture. A low arterial

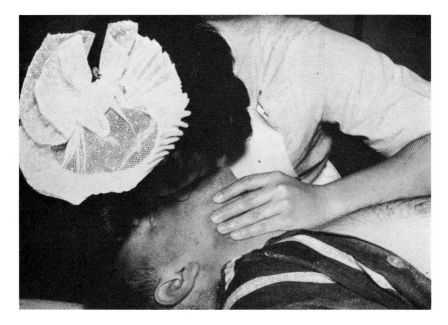

Fig. 14.6. Mouth to mouth respiration—the head and neck are extended and the position is maintained by a hand on the forehead which also pinches the nostrils. Ventilation is performed by placing the nurse's mouth completely over that of the patient and obtaining an airtight fit. The mouth is removed to allow the patient to exhale.

PO_2, respiratory and metabolic acidosis are thereby diagnosed and treated with increased ventilation or sodium bicarbonate infusion. The level of plasma potassium is also regularly monitored as it may vary markedly.

b. RESTORATION OF A NORMAL BEAT

If the nursing staff can achieve effective massage and ventilation the heart may restart before the arrival of the medical staff, and in any case they will have made the complete recovery of the patient more likely. Massage is continued while the rhythm is diagnosed, drugs given to increase the tone of the heart, and the appropriate action taken for the individual arrhythmia.

(i) CONTINUATION OF EXTERNAL MASSAGE AND VENTILATION

Ventilation is continued, usually with an endotracheal tube (Fig. 14.7). Frequently the upper airway has become soiled with secretions or vomit and requires aspiration before intubation. If the patient is conscious and struggling during external massage, nitrous oxide or other anaesthetic agent

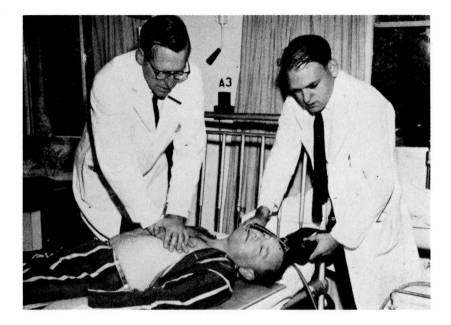

Fig. 14.7. The medical staff take over the performance of massage and ventilation. The anaesthetist intubates the patient and ventilates with oxygen from an anaesthetic trolley.

and curare (15 mg) or pancuronium are given to anaesthetize and paralyse the patient.

Even after the heart has been restored to a normal rhythm, a further period of massage may be necessary to sustain the blood pressure until the myocardium has recovered sufficiently to maintain the circulation.

(ii) DIAGNOSIS OF THE ABNORMAL RHYTHM

If it is not already connected, an electrocardiograph or oscilloscope is connected to the patient in order to diagnose whether the arrest is due to asystole, ventricular fibrillation or extreme bradycardia or tachycardia (Fig. 14.8). Asystole is shown as a straight line on the oscilloscope (Fig. 14.2), ventricular fibrillation as totally irregular waves (Fig. 14.3).

(iii) DRUGS

An intravenous infusion is started for fluid or blood replacement and as a channel for intravenous medications. The dilated external jugular vein is often the most convenient vein for cannulation. Rarely, if no intravenous drip can be quickly set up, injection of drugs can be made directly into the left ventricle by inserting a long fine needle over the probable position of the apex beat, directing it at 30° to the horizontal towards the second right costal

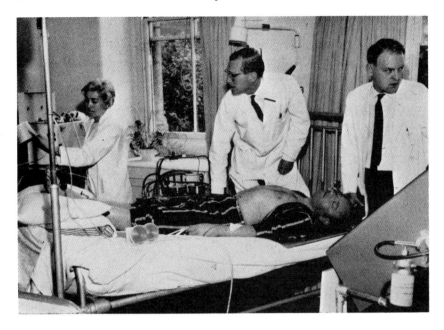

Fig. 14.8. The surgeon pauses briefly while the rhythm is determined on the electrocardiograph. If ventricular fibrillation is demonstrated, the anaesthetist adjusts the electric defibrillator.

cartilage. Finding the left ventricular cavity in a collapsed patient without an apical impulse is difficult and intracardiac injection often causes more trouble from pneumothorax, tamponade or coronary artery damage than it is worth. Injection of drugs into the dilated jugular veins is safer.

Regardless of the type of rhythm, certain drugs (see Table 14.1) are almost always used as a part of treatment. Sodium bicarbonate is given to counteract the metabolic acidosis that may have occurred while the circulation was arrested, although immediate and effective external massage prevents any important degree of acidosis developing. The amount of bicarbonate given will therefore depend on the effectiveness of the massage, and the length of time the patient is known to have been without a circulation, but is best checked by immediate measurement of pH and $P\text{CO}_2$ if facilities are available (page 105). If in doubt, 80 mmol is given initially followed by 40 mmol every quarter of an hour.

Myocardial stimulants, such as adrenaline and calcium chloride, increase the tone of the arrested heart or coarsen ventricular fibrillation prior to defibrillation. Isoprenaline, dopamine or Aramine may be used to sustain the blood pressure once the heart has restarted. All these drugs, in their correct strengths and volumes, are drawn up into labelled syringes under the direction of the anaesthetist while cardiac massage is continuing.

Table 14.1.

Drugs

Sodium bicarbonate (8.4% solution) for injection	
Calcium chloride 20% (hydrated)	5 ml
Adrenaline 1 : 10 000	10 ml
Lignocaine 1%	10 ml
Isoprenaline 0.01 mg in 1 ml	
Aramine or other vasopressor drug	

(iv) ASYSTOLE

Asystole may revert to sinus rhythm with a sharp blow on the chest or the start of cardiac massage. It is treated initially by giving calcium chloride (5ml of 20% solution, 0.5 g). If there is no response, adrenaline (10 ml of 1 : 10 000 or 1 ml of 1 : 1000 solution) is also given.

Sudden asystole may complicate the postoperative course of patients who have undergone certain operations which are particularly liable to complete heart block (tricuspid valve replacement, ostium primum atrial or ventricular septal defect). Such asystole is due to the acute onset of atrio-ventricular dissociation rather than myocardial mischief and is best treated by pacemaking, either externally or internally. If wires have been left in the right ventricle of such patients prophylactically at surgery, they will have been connected to an external pacemaker. Treatment of asystole merely involves switching the pacemaker on, checking however that an effective pulse is being produced. If no pulse is palpable, cardiac massage is begun and the full regime for cardiac arrest instituted.

(v) VENTRICULAR FIBRILLATION

Ventricular fibrillation is diagnosed by an irregular wavy line on the oscilloscope and the character of the fibrillation is important in planning treatment. If the fibrillation is coarse, particularly if it has been of only a few minutes' duration, a DC shock is applied immediately. Electrodes of the defibrillator are coated with electrode jelly and one placed at the base with the other over the apex of the heart (Fig. 14.9). 100–400 joules are given, with all personnel standing clear. Cardiac massage is then continued until a spontaneous pulse is elicited.

The closer the oscilloscopic trace of the ventricular fibrillation approximates to a flat line, i.e. the finer it is, the less likely is defibrillation to be successful. The tone of the myocardium is therefore improved with intravenous injections of adrenaline (10 ml of a 1 : 10 000 solution) and calcium (5 ml of 20% calcium chloride, 0·5 g), continued massage ensuring their entering the coronary circulation, A DC counter-shock is then administered. The cycle is repeated as necessary.

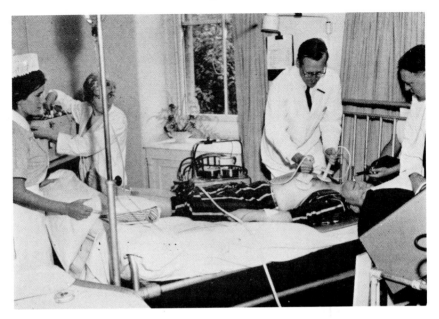

Fig. 14.9. Electrical defibrillation. The electrodes covered with electrode jelly are placed on the apex and base of the heart and a direct current (80–200 joules) passed. Everyone except the surgeon stands clear at the moment of discharge.

If the defibrillation is initially successful but then the rhythm reverts to ventricular fibrillation, 25 mg of lignocaine are given intravenously, followed by an infusion of 2 mg/minute. Disopyramide (Rythmodan), quinidine and procaineamide are tried if lignocaine fails to prevent recurrence (page 86). If all these measures fail, 100 ml of 50% dextrose containing 10 u insulin and 10 mmol potassium chloride are infused rapidly. If the serum potassium level is over 4.5 mmol/l, the potassium is omitted.

(vi) EXTREME BRADYCARDIA AND TACHYCARDIA
Extreme bradycardia is treated as asystole, extreme tachycardia as ventricular fibrillation.

(vii) FAILURE TO RESTART THE HEART
Failure to restart the heart may be due to hypoxia of the myocardium, hypothermia or irreversible cardiac damage. If efficient external massage and defibrillation fail to restart the heart, opening the chest is unlikely to be successful either but may be attempted. Thoracotomy does have one positive advantage in that unsuspected tamonade is excluded.

One member of the team quickly scrubs and dons gown and gloves, while another continues external massage. Rapid skin preparation and application

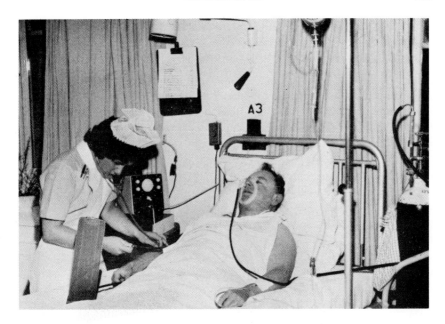

Fig. 14.10. Aftercare: continuous monitoring of pulse, blood pressure and ECG. Oxygen is administered by facemask. The urinary catheter is not seen.

of a large thoracotomy towel render the field sterile and massage is continued while the second member scrubs and reopens the operation wound or makes an incision in the 4th left interspace. The ribs are spread apart and the ventricles held between thumb and fingers and rhythmically massaged sufficiently firmly to produce a carotid pulse. If this can be managed without opening the pericardium, the myocardium will be somewhat protected from direct trauma but it is usually necessary to open it to produce an effective pulse. Injections of adrenaline and calcium, if they have not already been given, can be made directly into the left ventricle and massaged into the coronary arteries. Internal defibrillation is performed if necessary with electrodes applied directly to the myocardium and using a DC current of 40–80 joules. When the heart has restarted, the anaesthetist will have to anaesthetize the patient who may otherwise become conscious. The chest is then closed, leaving the pericardium widely open. All bleeding points arc secured and antibiotic powder sprinkled into each layer of the wound.

In spite of all measures, an effective cardiac contraction may not be achieved. The decision to abandon unsuccessful cardiac massage is a difficult one. Persistently fixed and dilated pupils suggest uncorrectable cerebral damage, and a toneless heart, totally unresponsive to touch after prolonged massage and injection of drugs, suggests that resuscitation is unlikely.

C. AFTERCARE AND TREATMENT OF COMPLICATIONS

Following resuscitation, the pulse, blood pressure and venous pressure are charted regularly and the usual measures for treatment of cardiac failure instituted if necessary (Fig. 14.10). Oxygen is administered with a facemask, or by mechanical ventilation if spontaneous respiration is inadequate. This is checked by blood gas analysis. The ECG oscilloscope monitors the cardiac rhythm, as further episodes of dysrhythmia or arrest may occur.

Inhalation of vomit is a common complication after cardiac arrest and the stomach is therefore aspirated by a nasogastric tube, which is left in position if stomach contents are considerable. A urinary catheter is also passed and the hourly urine output used as a measure of the cardiac output and to recognize oliguria if it occurs.

Immediate assessment of the cerebral state is made. If it has deteriorated as compared with the level before cardiac arrest, a corticosteroid such as dexamethasone may limit cerebral oedema (Chapter 11). Cardiac arrest is one of the few conditions following which cerebral dehydrating agents, such as mannitol, are useful because oedema tends to complicate cerebral anoxia.

Metabolic acidosis is assessed by analysing a sample of arterial blood. If it is present, it is corrected by the appropriate quantity of sodium bicarbonate (Chapter 7).

REFERENCES

ADGEY A.A.J. (1978) Electrical energy requirements for ventricular defibrillation. *Brit. Heart J.* **40**, 1197.

ALLEN J.D., PANTRIDGE J.F. & SHANKS R.G. (1971) Effects of lignocaine, propranolol and bretylium on ventricular fibrillation threshold. *Amer. J. Cardiol.* **28**, 555.

Brit. med. J. (1969) Complications of cardiac massage, **1**, 68.

CAMERATA S.J., WEIL M.H., HANASHIRO P.K. & SHUBIN H. (1971) Cardiac arrest in the cortically ill. *Circulation* **44**, 688.

GERBODE F. (1962) Cardiac arrest and resuscitation in *Surgery of the Chest*, ed. J.H. Gibbons, p. 166. Saunders, Philadelphia.

GILSTON A. (1965) Clinical and biochemical effects of cardiac resuscitation. *Lancet* **ii**, 1039.

JOHNSON A.L., TANSER P.H., ULAN R.A. and WOOD T.E. (1967) Results of cardiac resuscitation in 552 patients. *Amer. J. Cardiol.* **20**, 831.

JUDE J.R., KOUWENHOVEN W.B. & KNICKERBOCKER G.G. (1964) External cardiac massage. *Monogr. surg. Sci.* **1**, 59.

LOWN B., NEUMAN J., AMARASINGHAM R. & BERKOVITS B.V. (1962) Comparison of alternating current with direct electroshock across the closed chest. *Amer. J. Cardiol.* **10**, 223.

MILSTEIN B.B. (1963) Cardiac arrest and resuscitation. Lloyd Luke (Medical Books), London.

PAASKE F., HANSEN J.P.H., KOUDAHL G. & OLSEN J. (1968) Complications of closed chest cardiac massage in a forensic autopsy material. *Dan. med. Bull.* **15**, 225.

STEPHENSON H.E. (1964) Cardiac arrest and resuscitation, 2nd ed. Mosby, St Louis.
STEWART J.S.S. (1964) Management of cardiac arrest with special reference to metabolic acidosis. *Brit. med. J.* **2**, 476.
ZOLL P.M. (1971) Rational use of drugs for cardiac arrest and after cardiac resuscitation. *Amer. J. Cardiol.* **27**, 645.

CHAPTER 15

Infection

With the improvements over recent years in myocardial preservation during surgery, the foremost complication of cardiac surgery, the low cardiac output syndrome, has become markedly less frequent. As a result the main causes of prolonged hospital stay, morbidity and mortality today have become haemorrhage and infection, with the former proceeding not infrequently to the latter.

Patients who have undergone cardiac surgery have more disastrous complications from infection than other surgical patients. In general, postoperative infection is more likely in patients whose wounds have been open a long time, who have a low cardiac output, who have been hypothermic or in whom extracorporeal circulation has been used. Such patients are commonly the subjects of cardiac surgery today.

1. Infecting Organisms

Any organism may contaminate the wounds and tracheostomy site of the postoperative cardiac patient. Endocarditis after valve replacement has been shown to be often due to staphylococci—sometimes coagulase negative in type—or to fungi, particularly Candida.

2. Route of Entry

Infection appearing in the postoperative period has often been introduced on the operating table, but infection is still a danger in the intensive care unit and ward after operation unless strict precautions are taken. Infection comes from sources similar to those in the operating theatre.

a. FROM THE AIR

Infection by airborne organisms occurs if there is a high bacterial count in the air due to inadequate air changes in the ventilation system of the unit or infected patients in the unit.

b. DIRECT CONTACT

Organisms can be transferred from doctors' and nurses' clothing and fingers or infected equipment and bedding. Infection from the patient's own skin may occur, particularly with coagulase negative staphylococci.

c. INTRAVENOUS CATHETERS OR FLUID

Intensive care necessarily involves arterial and venous pressure monitoring, blood sampling and intravenous fluid and drug therapy. Indwelling intravenous plastic cannulae are essential for these purposes and they may remain in position for days or even weeks. These catheters are important causes of septicaemia. Relatively avirulent Gram-negative organisms are often responsible. The incidence of septicaemia increases if the lines are used for sampling instead of merely for infusions. Frequent disconnections and connections, 3-way tap adjustments and flushing of catheters are however necessary concomitants of such lines in intensive care units. Arterial pressure monitoring lines with sleeves of fibrin forming around them are particularly prone to contamination, as is the fluid used for flushing if left in position too long. Some organisms can travel up to 150 cm in 24 hours even against a pressure head, so that contamination of pressure transducers is dangerous even though they may be separated from the patient by a long length of tubing. Even disposable pressure transducer heads have become contaminated. Infection is more likely if blood, rather than electrolyte solution, is being used. Any bottle of blood may have become contaminated with bacteria at some point during preparation, collecting or storage and there will always be an incidence of transmission of viruses due to the blood donor having suffered from virus infection.

3. Prevention of Infection

Prevention of infection is important during and after cardiac surgery because treatment is often ineffective, particularly if prosthetic material has been used.

a. BEFORE SURGERY

The patient is washed in antiseptic (e.g. Chlorhexidine skin cleanser Hibiscrub) baths in an attempt to reduce skin infection. A nasal antiseptic (e.g. Naseptin) helps to eliminate staphylococci from the nose. Operations are postponed if an upper respiratory tract infection is present. Removal of all suspect teeth reduces the risk of postoperative bacterial endocarditis.

b. DURING SURGERY

The bacterial content of the air in the theatre is kept at as low a level as possible by reducing the number of people and movement to a minimum and by having frequent air changes in the ventilation system. Removing all staphylococcal carriers is usually impracticable because so many nurses and doctors are carriers and attempts to eliminate organisms may produce resistant strains. Regular checks for carriers are therefore usually not worth while, but skin sepsis, such as boils or exfoliative skin conditions, in theatre staff disperses large numbers of staphylococci which may easily infect the patient.

Direct contamination from the surgeon is avoided by careful scrubbing with antiseptic soaps (e.g. Hibiscrub, Betadine), wearing gowns that wrap around the back and sterile masks that are impervious to organisms. Gloves and superficial drapes are changed immediately before the intracardiac procedure itself. Instruments are packed and sterilized centrally. Endo-tracheal tubes, suction catheters and ventilators are sterilized before the start of each operation. The use of blood infected with serum or infective hepatitis is avoided as far as possible by screening donors for Australia antigen.

c. AFTER SURGERY

Early diagnosis and treatment of clinical infections are facilitated by regular bacterial cultures from the patient's sputum, urine and ventilator. Environmental surveys of the intensive care unit rarely yield useful information unless there is an outbreak.

(i) AIRBORNE INFECTION

Multiple air changes and isolation of contaminated patients reduces the bacterial content of the air in the intensive care unit to a minimum. Side rooms that have been used for heavily infected patients require thorough cleaning and the use of an appropriate disinfectant for surfaces, hand basins etc. White coats should be left outside the unit but masks, gowns and overshoes are generally considered to be bacteriologically unnecessary. The use of disposable plastic aprons by all staff and close attention of hand washing with chlorhexidine skin cleanser before passing from one patient to the next is more effective in preventing infection (Fig. 15.1). Doctors, nurses and visitors with upper respiratory tract or skin infections should be vigorously excluded from the unit.

(ii) INTRAVENOUS FLUIDS

Plastic catheters in veins are changed to a fresh site approximately every two days to avoid phlebitis and the risks of bacteraemia. Indwelling intravenous lines, 3-way taps, transducer heads and other pressure monitoring devices must be recognised as being potentially dangerous due to infection. A high

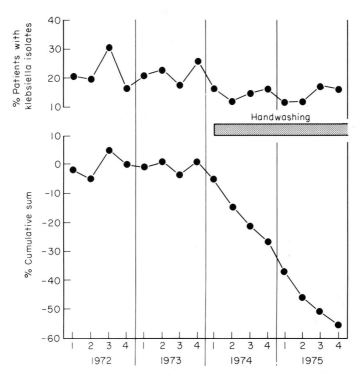

Fig. 15.1. The fall in the cumulative sum of patients with *Klebsiella* isolates associated with handwashing in an intensive therapy unit. (Reproduced by permission of the Editor of the *British Medical Journal* from Casewell *et al* 1977.)

standard of general cleanliness is required. All pressure monitoring equipment is sterilized between cases and at regular intervals in the same long-term patient—ethylene oxide, glutaraldehyde or disposable heads are used, remembering that glutaraldehyde may be injected into the vascular system inadvertently and cause permanent damage to vessels. Disposable transducers are also not immune to contamination. Sterile techniques are used when changing drip sets and bottles, drawing blood samples and calibrating transducers. All side ports in the intravenous system are treated as sterile. Blood is kept at 4°C and not allowed to stand in a warm room or remain connected to the patient for more than five hours because contaminating bacteria may then multiply more rapidly in it. Some bacteria may in fact multiply at 4°C. Plasma is used with caution and plasma substitutes preferred. Hepatitis B and 'non-B' are now the major risks from repeated plasma or blood infusions.

(iii) WOUND INFECTION
Wounds are kept dry, either exposed or covered with absorbent dressings that allow air to pass freely, except if a tracheostomy is done above a median

sternotomy when the upper end of the incision is covered with a waterproof dressing to prevent infected matter running down into the wound.

(iv) RESPIRATORY INFECTION

If artificial ventilation is employed, a no-touch technique is used for sucking out the airways (Fig. 7.5). The nurse wears a mask and uses a fresh sterile catheter each time, handling it with forceps or disposable gloves. Sterile water is used for humidification of oxygen and is put into sterile humidifying containers at the start of each case. Artificial ventilators and oxygen tents are disinfected between patients, and a fresh disposable face mask is used for each patient breathing spontaneously.

(v) URINARY INFECTION

Sterile connecting tubing is used to avoid infection passing up the plastic urinary catheter which is removed as soon as is practicable.

(vi) PROPHYLACTIC ANTIBIOTICS

Prophylactic antibiotics are used with the object of preventing wound infection and bacterial endocarditis after cardiac surgery although statistical evaluation of small series of patients with relatively low doses of antibiotics does not make a conclusive case for their use. The antibiotic chosen for prophylaxis should be active against a common cause of postoperative endocarditis, namely coagulase-negative staphylococci, and serious substernal sepsis with *Staphylococcus pyogenes*. Intramuscular cloxacillin or flucloxacillin with the premedication is commonly prescribed in this country and 500 mg of flucloxacillin given intramuscularly for at least two days postoperatively is appropriate. Some surgeons continue for five days, but there is no evidence that this is any better than two. Inclusion of gentamicin in the prophylaxis has the advantage of a spectrum that may include cloxacillin-resistant coagulase-negative staphylococci, but it also causes a greater disturbance of the patient's normal flora, and may thus promote emergence of infection with gentamicin-resistant organisms in the postoperative period or later. Vancomycin is one rational choice for patients that are hypersensitive to penicillins. Another possibility is a cephalosporin, but the one selected should have a good stability to staphylococcal α-lactamase. Tracheostomy sites invariably become colonized with bacteria, which are often opportunistic Gram-negative bacilli. Active clinical infection is uncommon and isolation of an organism is not an indication *per se* for antibiotic therapy.

4. Differential Diagnosis of Pyrexia

Pyrexia is common after any form of cardiac surgery and is almost invariable after extracorporeal circulation. This initial pyrexia usually resolves within 3–4 days.

Pyrexia may recur or persist beyond this time. The investigation of this pyrexia includes white and differential blood counts, Paul Bunnell test, blood, urine and wounds swab culture, cytomegalovirus titre, liver function tests and transaminase levels. The incident of pyrexia and raised white blood cell count bears, however, no statistically significant relation to overt infection.

a. ENDOCARDITIS FOLLOWING VALVE REPLACEMENT

Endocarditis may occur after any intracardiac operation as there is usually residual turbulence or nonabsorbable material left in contact with blood. The incidence of endocarditis is higher however after the implantation of artificial valves—prosthetic, homograft or xenograft—than after other operations because of the amount of foreign material. Postoperative endocarditis falls into two distinct categories depending on whether it begins before or after three months from the time of surgery.

(i) EARLY ONSET ENDOCARDITIS

Endocarditis within the first three months following surgery presents clinically with an acute septicaemic patient. The patient is ill, toxic and pyrexial (Fig. 15.2). The septicaemic patient may be markedly vasodilated with a large cardiac output (up to 10 l/min) and low arterial and venous pressures. Alternatively, the patient may be vasoconstricted with an unexplained low cardiac output. A third presentation may be as a consumptive coagulopathy. In view of this diversity of clinical presentations, endocarditis should be suspected in any patient who deteriorates following valve replacement.

The blood cultures are persistently positive and the organism can be recovered from valve vegetations at post mortem or at reoperation. The

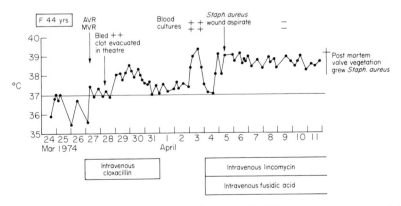

Fig. 15.2. Endocarditis on prosthetic valve 1 week following surgery caused by *Staphylococcus aureus*.

organism is usually *Staphylococcus aureus* of which the most likely source is a wound infection which may be clinically minor but from which the staphylococcus can be grown. Other organisms—*Pseudomonas, Candida, Staphylococcus albus* and rarer organisms—are sometimes responsible. Bacteraemia *per se* does not necessarily mean that the patient has endocarditis and bacteraemic patients who recover on antibiotics probably do not have endocarditis.

True early onset endocarditis has a bad prognosis with a mortality of 80% or more in spite of treatment. The high mortality of postoperative endocarditis demands effective prevention of which the most important is the elimination of wound infection.

(ii) LATE ONSET ENDOCARDITIS

Endocarditis occurring late on prosthetic heart valves is usually due to the same organisms that affect valves de novo. Most commonly the *Streptococcus viridans* is responsible, with *Staphylococcus albus, aureus, Brucella* and other organisms less commonly involved. The onset is subacute with the likely source of the organism being the mouth and teeth. The prognosis, once it has been diagnosed and effective antibiotics begun, is relatively good and is the same as that of endocarditis affecting rheumatic or degenerative valves. If valve malfunction or leak occurs, valve replacement is indicated.

There is no agreement as to how long antibiotics should be continued after endocarditis affecting prosthetic valves. Recurrences have been reported if antibiotics are not continued for six months but it is the usual practice to continue antibiotics for six weeks from the last positive blood culture and then to reassess the situation.

b. THE POSTPERFUSION SYNDROME (atypical mononucleosis syndrome)

This is probably due to cytomegalovirus infection of the fresh blood used at surgery. It presents with fever, characteristically at three to five weeks after operation, with enlargement of the spleen and monocytosis in which the abnormal cells have an abundant vacuolated cytoplasm. The patient is usually asymptomatic. Slight enlargement of the liver and lymph nodes may occasionally be associated. It is benign and resolves spontaneously without treatment.

c. THE POSTPERICARDIOTOMY SYNDROME

This may occur after any pericardial insult due to sterile inflammation of the pericardium and pleura, perhaps as a result of the development of antiheart antibodies or viral infection. The full syndrome consists of fever occurring one to three weeks after surgery, precordial and shouldertip pain, a raised jugular venous pressure, pericardial and pleural friction rubs, and enlargement of the cardiac shadow due to pericardial effusion on chest x-ray, but often only one or two of these features are present. It may recur months after operation.

d. HAEMOLYTIC ANAEMIA

Haemolytic anaemia may also cause pyrexia. It tends to follow the use of prosthetic material, particularly valves, though accelerated destruction of red cells follows all extracorporeal circulation. Its diagnosis is considered on page 166.

e. OTHER CAUSES OF PYREXIA

Causes of pyrexia unrelated to cardiac surgery have constantly to be borne in mind. Malaria is sought in patients from the tropics: venous thrombosis causes fever that resolves on ligation of leg veins: abdominal surgical emergencies, such as appendicitis, occur and are easily missed in the general postoperative wound discomfort, and pancreatitis may complicate low cardiac output states.

5. Treatment of Infection

a. WOUND

Once obvious clinical infection develops in the wound, scrutiny of recent bacteriological reports may indicate the infecting organism and its sensitivity. However, local clearance of pus including opening the wound and removing sutures that have stitch sinuses, is of prime importance. Irrigation of infected wounds has been a major advance in recent years in the prevention of serious complications of wound infections, such as suture line dehiscence. Insertion of a catheter to the extent of the wound sinus, with frequent irrigation with saline and Noxyflex, washes out all purulent discharge and accelerates resolution.

b. ENDOCARDITIS

Large doses of antibiotics are given on the advice of the department of microbiology directed at the specific organism. While cultures are being carried out, a possible combination of drugs is gentamicin and benzyl penicillin. If there is not a prompt resolution of pyrexia and improvement in the patient's general and cardiac state, particularly if there are signs of valve malfunction or leak, surgery is considered. Removal of the infected valve, taking care to send it for culture, is sometimes effective (Fig. 15.3).

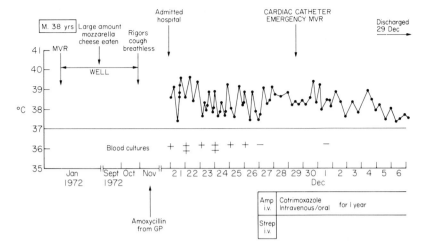

Fig. 15.3. Endocarditis on prosthetic valve 10 months following surgery caused by *Brucella melitensis*.

c. CHEST AND URINE

Maintaining clear bronchi by means of physiotherapy, avoiding retention of urine and appropriate antibiotic therapy minimize infection.

d. POSTPERICARDIOTOMY SYNDROME

Soluble aspirin, 600 mg four times a day, is effective in the treatment of the postpericardiotomy syndrome and is used by the author routinely for its anti-inflammatory activity in all undiagnosed postoperative pyrexia.

REFERENCES

AMOURY R.A., BOWMAN F.O. & MALM J.R. (1966) Endocarditis associated with intracardiac prostheses. *J. thorac. cardiovasc. Surg.* **51**, 36.

BRAIMBRIDGE M.V. (1969) Cardiac surgery and bacterial endocarditis. *Lancet* **i**, 1307.

BROWN A.H., BRAIMBRIDGE M.V., PANAGOPOULOS P. & SABAR E.F. (1969) The complications of median sternotomy. *J. thorac. cardiovasc. Surg.* **58**, 189.

CARLSTROM G., BELFRAGE S., OHLSSON N-M. & SWEDBERG J. (1968) Cytomegalovirus infection complicating open heart surgery. *Scand. J. thorac. cardiovasc. Surg.* **2**, 57.

CASEWELL M. & PHILLIPS I. (1977) Hands as a route of transmission of *Klebsiella* species. *Brit. med. J.* **2**, 1315.

CAUL E.D., CLARKE S.K.R., MOTT M.G., PERHAM T.G.M. & WILSON R.S.E. (1971) Cytomegalovirus infections after open heart surgery. *Lancet* **i**, 777.

CONWAY N., KOTHARI M.L., LOCKEY E. & YACOUB M.H. (1968) Candida endocarditis after heart surgery. *Thorax* **23**, 353.

DAYTON S. & PEARCE M.L. (1968) Cytomegalovirus infection following extracorporeal circulation. *Lancet* **ii**, 1298.

ENGLE M.E. & ITO T. (1961) The postpericardiotomy syndrome. *Amer. J. Cardiol.* **7**, 73.

EYKYN S.J. & BRAIMBRIDGE M.V. (1977) Open heart surgery complicated by postoperative malaria. *Lancet* **ii**, 411.

FEKETY F.R., CLUFF L.E., SABISTON D.C., SEIDL L.G., SMITH J.W. & THOBURN R. (1969) A study of antibiotic prophylaxis in cardiac surgery. *J. thorac. cardiovasc. Surg.* **57**, 757.

FIROR W.B. (1967) Infection following open-heart surgery, with special reference to the role of prophylactic antibiotics. *J. thorac. cardiovasc. Surg.* **53**, 371.

FONG I.W., BAKER C.B. & MCKEE D.C. (1979) The value of prophylactic antibiotics in aorta-coronary bypass operations. *J. thorac. cardiovasc. Surg.* **78**, 908.

GOODMAN J.S., SCHAFFNER W., COLLINS H.A., BATTERSBY E.J. & KOENIG M.G. (1968) Infection after cardiovascular surgery: clinical study including examination of antimicrobial prophylaxis. *New England J. med.* **278**, 117.

HERR R., STARR A., MCCORD C.W. & WOOD J.A. (1965) Special problems following valve replacement: embolus, leak, infection and red cell damage. *Ann. thorac. Surg.* **1**, 403.

KAHN D.R., ERTEL P.Y., MURPHY W.H., KIRSH M.M., VATHAYANON S., STERN A.M. & SLOAN H. (1967) Pathogenesis of the postpericardiotomy syndrome. *J. thorac. cardiovasc. Surg.* **54**, 682.

MCGUINESS J.B. & TAUSSIG H.B. (1962) The postpericardiotomy syndrome. *Circulation* **26**, 500.

MAHALU W. & BRAIMBRIDGE M.V. (1979) Cardiac valve replacement and endocarditis. *Proc. Assoc. Surgeons East Africa* **2**, 152.

MILLER D.R., MURPHY K. & CESARIO T. (1978) Pseudomonas infection of the sternum and costal cartilages. *J. thorac. cardiovasc. Surg.* **76**, 723.

NELSON J.C. & NELSON R.M. (1967) The incidence of hospital wound infection in thoracotomies. *J. thorac. cardiovasc. Surg.* **54**, 586.

OCHSNER J.L., MILLS N.L. & WOOLVERTON W.C. (1972) Disruption and infection of the median sternotomy incision. *J. thorac. cardiovasc. Surg.* **13**, 394.

ROSES D.F., ROSE M.R. & RAPAPORT F.T. (1974) Febrile responses associated with cardiac surgery. *J. thorac. cardiovasc. Surg.* **67**, 251.

ROSS B. (1964) Pyrexia after heart surgery due to virus infection transmitted by blood transfusion. *Thorax* **19**, 159.

SHAFER R.S. & HALL W.H. (1970) Bacterial endocarditis following open heart surgery. *Amer. J. Cardiol.* **25**, 602.

SLAUGHTER L., MORRIS J.E. & STARR A. (1973) Prosthetic valve endocarditis: a twelve year review. *Circulation* **47**, 1319.

STONEY W.S., ALFORD W.C., BURRUS G.R., FRIST R.A. & THOMAS C.S. (1978) Median sternotomy dehiscence. *Ann. thorac. Surg.* **26**, 421.

VAN DER GELD H. (1964) Antiheart antibodies in the postpericardiotomy and the postmyocardial infarction syndromes. *Lancet* **ii**, 617.

WEINSTEIN R.A., JONES E.L., SCHWARZMANN S.W. & HATCHER C.R. JR (1976) Sternal osteomyelitis and mediastinitis after open heart operation: pathogenesis and prevention. *Ann. thorac. Surg.* **21**, 442.

CHAPTER 16

Special Problems of Postoperative Care in Infancy and Childhood

M. JONES & J. STARK

1. Introduction

At present, cardiac surgery in infants and small children has progressed to the extent that most lesions may be corrected early in life. In this chapter particular emphasis is placed on the special care of infants and children undergoing operations for congenital heart disease. In theory and in practice the postoperative management of infants and children is similar in most ways to that of adult patients but their potential for growth, their particular and often immature metabolic processes and the cardiovascular physiology of congenital malformations demand special consideration.

2. Preoperative Considerations

Many infants present critically ill or even moribund and postoperative results are profoundly influenced by the initial assessment, diagnostic evaluation and preparatory procedures.

On admission, enquiries are made about perinatal problems, about infant and maternal medication, gestational age (prematurity or dysmaturity), birth weight and method of feeding. 25% of children have associated anomalies other than the cardiac defect and these are looked for. All neonates less than 10 days old receive 1 mg of vitamin K parenterally.

Intensive care involves three distinct periods: before, during and after surgery. Intensive care is started, if possible, from the time diagnostic suspicion is raised, and continues during transport to hospital and admission, during diagnostic tests, including cardiac catheterization and angiocardiography and during the interval between the completion of these tests and the beginning of the operation. Continuous monitoring of the electrocardiogram and arterial and central venous pressures are instituted as soon as possible.

Endotracheal intubation and artificial ventilation may be necessary if an infant is hypoventilating. Body heat is best preserved in an incubator or with an overhead infra-red heater. Intensive care is continued throughout the operation and during the postoperative period.

BLOOD SAMPLES

Blood samples are taken for arterial blood gases, electrolytes, including calcium, and for glucose, haematological and coagulation indices, blood grouping and cross matching and, in coloured children and children of Mediterranean descent, for sickle cell traits. Obtaining adequate blood samples from small infants and from cyanotic children with marked polycythaemia can be a trying experience for the patient and for the person obtaining the sample. The femoral artery or vein is the site of first choice with radial, brachial or dorsalis pedis arteries available. The internal jugular vein can also be used, even in the smallest infants. It is important to use an aseptic technique. Arterial puncture is followed by pressure for ten minutes to prevent haematoma formation which will preclude further sampling from the same site as well as causing discomfort and a nidus for infection. Pressure on the artery should be sufficient to prevent bleeding from the puncture but insufficient to occlude the vessel completely. Larger or repeated samples of venous blood may be obtained by using a small needle of 'butterfly' type and attaching the aspirating syringe to the end of the 'butterfly' tubing. The necessity for manually stabilizing the needle in a small vein or artery is thereby obviated.

Blood samples can be taken from central venous or arterial lines should these have been inserted previously. The disadvantages of sampling from these lines are the necessity of clearing them after sampling with flushing solution in infants with small total fluid limits; haemolysis of the sample from rapid withdrawal through small calibre tubing; and artefacts in samples for clotting indices because the lines have usually been flushed with heparinized saline.

Complications of arterial and venepuncture include haematoma formation, septic arthritis from femoral punctures, and rarely reflex bradycardia or hypotension following vagal stimulation during internal jugular puncture.

Capillary samples are less reliable than those obtained by either of the above methods, the site of sampling being either a finger, toe or heel. A small stab incision is made after wiping the site with an antiseptic solution. The first drop or two of blood is wiped away and the sample is collected drop by drop in a capillary tube or small phial. If obtained from an extremity warmed to produce hyperaemia, capillary blood characteristics are similar to those of arterial blood but this may not be true in abnormal physiological states which occur during low cardiac output conditions. Other problems of using this method include the possibility of producing haemolysis or of having tissue fluid contaminate the sample.

3. Initial Postoperative Management

a. INITIAL MEASURES ON RETURN FROM THE OPERATING THEATRE

Those intimately responsible for the child need complete knowledge of the preoperative clinical problems and medication, such as preoperative low cardiac output, acidosis, hypoxaemia, electrolyte and haematological abnormalities, infection and state of nutrition. Note is taken of preoperative medication and when drugs were discontinued, particularly digitalis, diuretics, steroids, beta-blockers, salicylates and anticoagulants. The care of neonates requires consideration of maternal medication also.

On return to the intensive therapy unit (ITU) from the theatre, clinical assessment, respiratory stabilization and cardiovascular monitoring are established. The immediate measures on return to the ITU are basically similar to those in the adult (Chapter 2).

Arterial, atrial and central venous lines are connected to transducers and to the monitoring equipment and the child is connected to the ventilator. Staff that were present during the operation record for the ITU staff the following information:

1. Type of operative repair.
2. Post-correction intracardiac pressures.
3. Length of perfusion.
4. Type of myocardial preservation used and the length of aortic crossclamping.
5. Position of drains, pacing wires, atrial and other monitoring lines.
6. Size of the endotracheal tube, volume and inspired oxygen concentration (F_IO_2) used for ventilation.
7. Amount of urine excreted during the operation.
8. Any special comments

Fluid balance is critical in small infants. Because the total amount of intravenous fluid given per hour may be very small, slow infusion pumps are best both for fluid administration and for flushing arterial, atrial and venous monitoring lines. When calculating the fluid balance *all* fluid given, including that used for flushing monitoring lines and oral fluid given via a nasogastric tube, is recorded. Fluid output includes urine and nasogastric aspirate with diarrhoea or profuse sweating taken into account.

Chest drainage is replaced with whole blood or plasma to maintain a haematocrit (PCV) of 35–42% (haemoglobin of 12–14 g/100 ml) but transfusion in the immediate postoperative period is governed more by the level of the atrial pressures than by blood loss from chest drains.

Sedation is necessary, particularly in patients requiring ventilatory support and in agitated and confused children. Morphine sulphate in a dose of 0.1 mg/kg is given intravenously. Subsequent doses of 0.2 mg/kg are given at four hourly intervals if required. This can be supplemented by diazepam

(Valium) in i.v./i.m. doses of 0.1 mg/kg. Paralysing agents are rarely necessary (pancuronium 0.1 mg/kg intravenously in 1–2 hourly intervals). Routine sedation after the first 24 or 48 hours can be provided with trichloral in a dose of 30 mg/kg orally.

Parents require reassurance. They may experience guilt feelings because of having an abnormal child and they are concerned about their other children and loss of time from work in addition to genuine concern about the patient himself. Family visits, even for a few minutes, help to relieve anxiety and encourage cooperation of the child.

b. BASIC PROCEDURES

Postoperative care may be more difficult in neonates and infants than in adults and attention to detail is essential. In infants procedures are best performed with the patient under a radiant heat warmer which protects them against heat loss during the procedure and allows better access to them than an incubator. Constant observation of the general status of the patient is necessary during the performance of any of the basic procedures.

(i) MONITORING AND INFUSION LINES

Survival may depend upon adequate monitoring and infusion lines. Percutaneous placement of the lines is preferable because both early and late patency of the vessels is better than that following cut-down incisions and the risk of infection is less.

Sites for venous lines include the internal or external jugular vein, basilic vein or the saphenous vein at the groin and at the medial malleolus at the ankle. Umbilical vein cannulae may be used in neonates. The cannula is passed from the umbilical vein in the umbilical stump via the ductus venosus into the inferior vena cava. Using sterile operative techniques, the umbilical stump is amputated close to the abdominal wall using a scalpel. The vein is usually in the 12 o'clock position. The vein wall is held with the forceps and a radio-opaque catheter inserted—the distance for insertion being determined as two-thirds of the distance from the umbilicus to the mid-sternum, some 6–8 cm. With the cannula in the correct position, blood should be easily aspirated. The cannula is then secured by a suture and antibiotic ointment and a sterile dressing applied. Caution is taken if the umbilical catheter is used to administer hyperosmolar substances such as bicarbonate, THAM, or hypertonic glucose solution because infusion of these into the liver may cause hepatic necrosis.

The usual sites for percutaneous *arterial monitoring lines* are radial, brachial, femoral and dorsalis pedis arteries with the radial artery of a non-dominant hand preferred (Table 16.1). The size of the cannula varies from gauge 22 in small infants to gauge 20 in older children. If an arterial cut-down is necessary, the radial artery is again preferred. The length of the cannula is determined prior to insertion so that it passes no further than a third of the way from the wrist to the elbow. Air bubbles or clots are carefully excluded as they may be easily flushed into the central arterial circulation because the distance from the radial to the carotid artery is only 10–15 cm—less than 2 ml of fluid will clear this distance. Both arterial and venous lines may be positioned through a single ante-cubital incision, using the brachial artery and basilic vein.

An umbilical artery cannula may be used for arterial blood sampling and pressure monitoring. Using a procedure identical to that for umbilical vein cannulation, one of the two umbilical arteries (located at 4 and 8 o'clock) is identified and the radio-opaque cannula passed from the umbilical artery into the aorta, preferably above the ductus arteriosus. Returning blood should be pulsatile and arterialized. Its position should be confirmed by x-ray because a cannula below the diaphragm or beyond the aortic arch may allow infusions to pass in concentrated form directly into a visceral vessel or other small artery causing tissue necrosis. The timing and technique of removal of umbilical cannulae are important in children because of the risk of infection and subsequent portal vein thrombosis. The cannulae are removed within 23–28 hours. The suture is divided, the catheter removed and gentle pressure applied to the stump.

Left and right atrial monitoring lines are inserted through purse strings at the time of surgery directly into the atria. A pulmonary artery line may be inserted via the right ventricle. The knowledge of both atrial pressures helps in the assessment of cardiac performance and facilitates decisions about the correct preload (see page 39). The right atrial line can also be used for the infusion of catecholamines, estimation of mixed venous Po_2 and injection of dye or cold saline for cardiac output estimations. The pulmonary artery line can be removed slowly and any residual right ventricular outflow obstruction measured by a continual pressure trace taken during removal. The atrial and pulmonary artery lines are usually removed the day after surgery. There is a greater risk of bleeding than in adults and they are therefore removed before the chest drains. In infants intracardiac lines are never removed all at once. Cumulative bleeding of even 10–20 ml may be dangerous and it is best to remove the lines at about 30-minute intervals.

(ii) PACEMAKER WIRES
Temporary epicardial, atrial and ventricular pacemaker wires are left in position until the risk of dysrhythmias is minimal—usually 7–10 days after surgery—and are best removed at the time of removal of the skin sutures. If difficulty occurs in removing a wire, it is painted with antiseptic, severed at skin level while on traction and allowed to retract beneath the skin.

(iii) URINARY CATHETER
Urinary bladder catheters may pose problems in small patients. Because of

their small calibre, they are easily occluded by particulate matter in the urine or even by the lubricant used to insert them. Care is taken not to insert the catheter too far in an infant because the catheter coils, kinks and occludes. Small (6–8 French) catheters without retaining balloons are used in infants and are therefore more easily displaced than the Foley type catheters. A small feeding tube is also suitable for this purpose. Because the child's bladder is small and a child is less easily immobilized than an adult, trauma to the bladder and urethra may occur. Neonates and infants will usually pass urine following suprapubic massage which allows monitoring of urinary output without an indwelling catheter but a urinary catheter is desirable even in neonates for at least the first 24 hours.

Bladder aspiration is sometimes useful for obtaining urinary samples for culture without passing a catheter. As the infant's pelvis is small, the bladder is an intra-abdominal organ and may be safely aspirated. The patient should not have voided for an hour previously and the bladder should be palpable. The child is immobilized and a small 22 gauge needle with an attached syringe is inserted into the midline 1 or 2 cm above the symphysis pubis at an angle directed caudally. With gentle suction the urine is aspirated.

(iv) NASOGASTRIC TUBE

Nasogastric tubes are important to prevent gastric dilatation. It is safest to insert them in all children both after palliative and corrective cardiac operations. Infants are air swallowers and eructation of swallowed air is not possible in the sedated, unconscious or paralysed patient and infant endotracheal tubes have no inflatable cuffs to prevent aspiration of vomit. Nasogastric tubes are used also for postoperative gavage feedings, a technique especially useful for nutrition when prolonged ventilatory support is necessary.

4. Cardiovascular Problems

The principles of evaluation of the postoperative cardiovascular state of an infant or a child are similar to those of adults (Chapter 5), but special considerations are necessary in view of their size and age. Normal blood pressure depends on the age of the child (Table 16.1). Heart rate also varies according to age (Table 16.2).

The cardiac output should ideally be above $3.0 \, l/min/m^2$. The mean right atrial pressure varies from 1–5 mmHg and the left atrial pressure from 5–10 mmHg with zero estimated at mid-chest level (0–5 mmHg from the sternal angle). These atrial pressures (ventricular filling pressure or preload) may have to be raised to achieve an optimal cardiac output in the postoperative period and pressures as high as 15 mmHg may occasionally be required when there is residual ventricular outflow tract obstruction, reduced ventricular

Table 16.1. Normal blood pressure for various ages. From Nadas & Fyler (1972), courtesy of W. B. Saunders, Philadelphia.

Age (years)	Mean systolic $\pm 2SD$	Mean diastolic $\pm 2SD$
Newborn	80 ± 16	46 ± 16
6 months–1 year	89 ± 29	60 ± 10
2	99 ± 25	64 ± 25
4	99 ± 20	65 ± 20
5–6	95 ± 14	55 ± 9
8–9	105 ± 16	57 ± 9
11–12	113 ± 18	59 ± 10

compliance because of ventricular hypertrophy, or residual A–V valve and pulmonary vascular disease.

The urinary output is one of the best indirect indices of cardiac output. The minimal acceptable urinary output is 0.5 ml/kg/hr or 400 ml/m^2 in 24 hours but preferably should be more than 1 ml/kg/hr.

a. HEART RATE

The optimum heart rate (Table 16.2) is achieved, if it is too slow, with chronotropic drugs or electrically with pacing. Isoprenaline (0.03–0.16 μg/kg/min) may be administered via a microdrip. Atropine (0.01 mg/kg) is also sometimes useful. Pacing wires will have been placed in the atria

Table 16.2. Normal heart rates in infants and children. From Ziegler (1951), courtesy of Charles C. Thomas, Springfield, Illinois.

Age	Heart rate		
	Average	Minimum	Maximum
0–24 hours	125	88	166
1 day–1 week	138	100	188
1 week–1 month	162	125	188
1–3 months	161	115	215
3–6 months	147	125	215
6 months–1 year	147	115	188
1–3 years	130	100	188
3–5 years	105	68	150
5–8 years	102	75	150
8–12 years	88	51	125
12–16 years	83	38	125

and/or ventricles at the time of operation. Atrial pacing is preferable to ventricular pacing because of the beneficial effect of sinus rhythm but it is usually more difficult to achieve. A heart rate faster than the optimal is treated with digitalis or beta blockers. If it is due to supraventricular tachycardia or atrial fibrillation, DC countershock is considered.

b. PRELOAD (ATRIAL PRESSURES)

Patients with right heart obstructive lesions, including tetralogy of Fallot, pulmonary stenosis, pulmonary atresia, tricuspid atresia and pulmonary obstructive vascular disease require higher right atrial pressures (RA or CVP) than patients with a normal right heart. Patients with left heart obstructive lesions and hypertrophied, poorly compliant left ventricles require elevated left atrial pressures for optimal left ventricular preload.

Patients with tricuspid atresia after the Fontan operations (right atrial to pulmonary artery or right atrial to right ventricle conduit) are prone to develop right pleural effusions and hepatomegaly. In these patients, the right atrial pressure and signs of right heart failure have to be titrated against cardiac output.

Patients with transposition of the great arteries (ventriculo-arterial discordance, TGA) are discussed in terms of pressures in the pulmonary venous and systemic venous atria to prevent confusion. Following a Mustard operation, the pulmonary venous atrium may be poorly compliant because of the muscular inter-atrial septum, because of the non-contractile intra-atrial baffle and because of the enlargement of the pulmonary venous atrium with a non-contractile patch. The margin of error in judging preload requirements in these patients is therefore small, and both pulmonary congestion and pleural effusions may occur.

Patients who have had total anomalous pulmonary venous drainage repaired are prone to develop pulmonary congestion which may result in respiratory insufficiency. In these conditions the atrial pressure is kept as low as is compatible with an adequate cardiac output. Inadequate left and right heart syndromes may produce difficulties. Inadequate right hearts are most common in neonates with obstructive lesions of the right heart, pulmonary atresia, tricuspid atresia, congenital tricuspid stenosis and Ebstein's anomaly. Inadequate left hearts occur in some patients with congenital aortic stenosis, mitral stenosis, interrupted aortic arch and the hypoplastic left heart syndrome. Again in these conditions, the atrial pressure may have to be kept higher than normal.

A discussion of preload abnormalities would be incomplete without consideration of cardiac tamponade (Chapter 5). In small patients, the onset of tamponade may be particularly insidious. Only small volumes of blood or clot may compromise cardiovascular function in a small mediastinum. Often oliguria is the only presenting sign. Anticipation with prompt recognition and operation is essential if these patients are to be saved.

It should be mentioned that tamponade may occur even in patients who have had the pericardium removed, as in the Mustard operation for TGA. In this situation, the heart may be compressed by clot behind the sternum. Bleeding into the thymus gland also may cause acute compression of an external conduit, especially in small infants with persistent truncus arteriosus.

c. AFTERLOAD (VASCULAR RESISTANCE/IMPEDANCE)

The best method of relieving an abnormally elevated *right ventricular afterload* is to relieve completely right ventricular outflow tract obstruction. Relief is not always possible because of peripheral pulmonary stenosis, small branch pulmonary arteries, pulmonary vascular obstructive disease or residual left heart obstructive lesions. The pulmonary valve may be regurgitant due to operative incision, excision of valve leaflets, right ventricular outflow tract patches or valveless conduits across the pulmonary annulus. Such pulmonary regurgitation is worse when right ventricular afterload and pulmonary vascular resistance increase and the right ventricle suffers from both pressure and volume overload. Means for reducing the pulmonary vascular resistance include administering oxygen to avoid hypoxaemia, avoiding acidosis and reducing reactive pulmonary arteriolar constriction pharmacologically with isoprenaline, tolazoline or priscoline. Morphine and chlorpromazine may also decrease pulmonary artery pressure.

As on the right side, the ideal way to relieve left ventricular afterload is to relieve completely left ventricular outflow tract obstruction, but again this is not always possible. The main reason is that compromises are made by the surgeon because of reluctance to place prosthetic valves in children. Additional causes are a small aortic annulus or injury to the mitral valve or conducting mechanism by extensive resection. A major additional cause of increased left ventricular afterload is increased systemic resistance, usually due to arteriolar vasoconstriction. An elevated left heart afterload may or may not be accompanied by an elevated systemic blood pressure.

Acute alterations of cardiovascular physiology also occur following correction of mitral regurgitation, either as an isolated lesion or in combination with atrioventricular canal defects. Before correction the left ventricle faces a low afterload because it ejects partly into a low pressure chamber, the left atrium. After correction of the mitral regurgitation, the left ventricle may be unable to cope with even a normal systemic vascular resistance, particularly when associated with a left to right shunt. Optimal cardiac output and myocardial efficiency may demand the systemic afterload to be kept at normal or even below normal levels.

The opposite occurs in patients with dynamic types of left ventricular outflow tract obstruction such as lesions accompanied by disproportionate hypertrophy of the ventricular septum (obstructive cardiomyopathy, idiopathic hypertrophic subaortic stenosis). Muscular subaortic obstruction also occurs in combination with coarctation of the aorta and the parachute mitral valve syndrome. The important postoperative consideration with these lesions is that the left ventricular outflow tract obstruction and the gradient are inversely related to the systemic afterload—a diminished systemic afterload will actually increase the left ventricular outflow obstruction as its walls approximate more easily.

Excluding intra-aortic balloon counterpulsation (Chapter 5), methods for decreasing *systemic vascular resistance* are mainly pharmacological but warming the patient and eliminating shivering will produce peripheral vasodilatation, decreasing left ventricular afterload. Therapy is best begun by administering chlorpromazine intravenously in a dose of 0.1–0.3 mg/kg. Sodium nitroprusside is more effective, with an infusion rate of 0.2–2 μg/kg/min. Because of the possibility of cyanide poisoning (rare) the dose is not increased above 7 μg/kg/min and the infusion is discontinued within 48 hours. Decreasing the peripheral vascular resistance usually requires volume expansion, with the left and right heart filling pressures (preload) being kept constant by transfusion.

A spontaneously markedly increased cardiac output and decreased systemic vascular resistance are associated with septicaemia, even though pyrexia and rigors may be absent.

d. MYOCARDIAL CONTRACTILITY

If the heart rate, preload and afterload are optimally adjusted and the cardiac output is still inadequate, myocardial contractility has to be improved. Drugs to increase myocardial contractility include calcium, catecholamines, digitalis preparations, glucagon, hypertonic glucose and steroids. Caution is necessary in patients with congenital heart defects with an increased pulmonary arteriolar resistance, because many agents that increase myocardial contractility also have alpha-adrenergic effects upon the pulmonary vasculature and cause pulmonary vasoconstriction.

Calcium is a powerful inotropic agent, though its effect is transient. Decreased cardiac performance may occur due to transfused bank blood because of calcium binding by the citrate. Standard bolus intravenous doses are 0.25–1 mmol and doses of 0.1 mmol are given for each 100 ml of transfused blood, avoiding injection into lines containing citrated blood or bicarbonate. Caution must also be taken when giving calcium simultaneously with digitalis preparations as calcium may potentiate digitalis toxicity.

Currently the preferred choice of inotropic agent for intravenous infusion in children is *dopamine*, which has the advantage of increasing cardiac output and myocardial contractility while improving renal blood flow and urine

Table 16.3. Usual dosage of catecholamines

Drug	Solution	Dose μg/kg/min
Dopamine (Intropin)	6 mg/kg/in 100 ml	2–10
Isoproterenol (isoprenaline)	0.5–2 mg/100 ml	0.03–0.16
Epinephrine (adrenaline)	1–3 mg/100 ml	0.06–0.32

All drugs diluted in 5% dextrose. In newborns and small infants increased concentration may be required to avoid fluid overload.

output. It lowers systemic and probably pulmonary vasculature resistance with less tachycardia in low infusion doses (less than 10 μg/kg/min) than other inotropic infusions. Its effect upon reactive pulmonary hypertension has not been fully evaluated so that caution should be exercised when using dopamine in patients with pulmonary hypertension. The infusion is started with a dose of 2–3 μg/kg/min and increased as required, though a dose of 10 μg/kg/min is rarely exceeded* (Table 16.3).

Occasionally, *adrenaline* will be effective in increasing cardiac output when dopamine is not. The infusion rate for adrenaline is 0.06–0.32 μg/kg/min with a maximum of 1 μg/kg/min. *Isoprenaline* is also useful, but tends to cause unacceptable tachycardia in children. The infusion rate is 0.03–0.16 μg/kg/min.

Digitalis preparations are chronic agents which are not very suitable for administration in the immediate postoperative period, except for treatment of supraventricular tachycardias. If indicated, digoxin is started after the first 24–36 hours. This delay avoids creating confusion during the initial management of dysrhythmias and metabolic and electrolyte disturbances. There is a particular propensity for digitalis-induced dysrhythmias in patients with pulmonary hypertension and with right ventricular hypertrophy. The presumed mechanism is that hypoxia and acidosis potentiate digitalis intoxication.

e. SUBACUTE AND CHRONIC HEART FAILURE

The signs and symptoms of persistent cardiac failure after the first 48 hours include excessive weight gain, unexplained tachycardia, tachypnoea, hepatomegaly, ascites, and pulmonary congestion. Often the only sign of cardiac failure in infants may be poor feeding and general irritability. Severe cardiac failure early or late postoperatively usually means the presence of

* A solution of 6 mg/kg/body weight of dopamine in 100 ml of 5% dextrose is made. With a microdrip set (60 drops = 1 ml) one drop = 1 μg/kg/min which facilitates the calculations.

residual or recurrent defects or malfunctioning valvular prostheses. Early re-evaluation, cardiac catheterization and reoperation are considered. Today, with myocardial preservation with cardioplegia, severe postoperative cardiac failure in children is rarely due to irreversible myocardial damage.

(i) DIGITALIZATION

Digoxin is not given prophylactically: its use is reserved for patients with clinical cardiac failure. However, certain patients are likely to require it: those with residual defects or gradients, those who needed inotropic support early postoperatively, or those who have large right ventricular outflow tract patches. The regime for administering digoxin is illustrated on Table 16.4: note the difference between the parenteral and oral doses and also the smaller doses for the neonate and the small infant. Patients who were taking digoxin before operation, in whom it was stopped not more than 48 hours before the operation and who have normal renal function, are started on the maintenance dose postoperatively rather than the digitalizing dose.

To initiate digoxin administration, half of the total digitalizing dose is given at once, usually intravenously, a quarter after eight hours, and the remaining quarter 16 hours after the initial dose. When acutely digitalizing the patient, the electrocardiogram is observed before each dose for conduction disturbances, prolongation of the PR interval, direction of the P wave axis, and duration of the QRS complex. These values are compared with the normal for age and heart rate given in the subsection on rhythm disturbances

Table 16.4. Digoxin (Lanoxin, Burroughs Wellcome). Dose schedule for digitalization and maintenance

	Total digitalizing dose in 24 hours		Maintenance dose in 24 hours	
	Oral (mg/kg)	Parenteral (mg/kg)	Oral (mg/kg)	Parenteral (mg/kg)
Neonates and infants Less than 3.0kg	0.04	0.03	0.015	0.010
Infants (over 1 month) and children up to 2 years	0.06	0.04	0.025	0.015
Children 2–10 years	0.04	0.03	0.015	0.010
	Half the total dose is usually given at once, a quarter after 8 hours and the remaining quarter 8 hours later		Usually given as a divided dose twice and occasionally three times daily.	

For convenience of oral administration, each dose should be 'rounded off' to the nearest 0.01 mg and pacemakers. In addition to rhythm disturbances, digitalis toxicity is suspected in any child who is vomiting. The serum potassium is also checked before each dose during the digitalization process. Maintenance digoxin doses (one half of the daily dose given in Table 16.4) are administered twice daily.

Serum digoxin levels aid digitalis administration in patients with malabsorption, renal dysfunction or rhythm disturbances. It should be pointed out that the sample should be taken at least 6 hours after the last dose of digoxin when the child has been on a stable dose for 48 hours. Serum digoxin levels are especially helpful in these circumstances, since poor feeding and vomiting may be manifestations of toxicity. One suspects digitalis toxicity if the serum digoxin levels are greater than 2.7 ng/ml, although infants may have levels as high as 4.0 ng/ml without clinical evidence of toxicity.

(ii) DIURETICS
Fluid restriction is preferable to diuretic therapy in the treatment of the milder forms of postoperative fluid retention because of the tendency for diuretics to produce electrolyte abnormalities, particularly hypokalaemia. It is usually however impracticable to restrict fluids to more than one-third to one-half of maintenance requirements. A liquid diet provides most of an infant's or a small child's calories; therefore, severe fluid restriction is detrimental to clinical recovery. If fluid restriction alone is inadequate, the preferred diuretic agent is frusemide (Lasix) given in doses of 0.5–2.0 mg/kg parenterally or orally. Doses of up to 5.0 mg/kg may be given for severe, intractable failure. Occasionally, ethacrynic acid is effective when frusemide is not. The dose of ethacrynic acid is 0.5–1.0 mg/kg intravenously. The addition of oral spironolactone may be also useful (6.25 mg 8 hourly in infants and 12.5 mg 8 hourly in older children).

Sodium restriction is of benefit in treating postoperative subacute and chronic cardiac failure and low sodium milk formulas are available. Older children are best managed using a 'no added salt' diet, which is a diet to which no additional salt is added in the cooking or at the table, and one which excludes obviously salty foods.

f. RHYTHM DISTURBANCES AND PACEMAKERS

In general most rhythm disturbances after operation are treated in a similar manner and with the same pharmacological agents as in adults. A discussion of specific dysrhythmias will not therefore be undertaken here. Heart rates and blood pressures vary with age, as do electrocardiographic measurements, and it is necessary to take into consideration the patient's age and heart rate when examining the PR interval.

Rhythm disturbances and conduction abnormalities occur as part of the natural history of some congenital cardiac defects. These rhythm problems include complete heart block in congenitally corrected transposition of the great arteries (atrioventricular discordance, ventriculo-arterial discordance) and tachyarrhythmias in Ebstein's anomaly and the pre-excitation syndromes (Wolff–Parkinson–White syndrome). Patients with cardiac malpositions, situs abnormalities and congenitally corrected transposition of the great arteries frequently have abnormal PR intervals and abnormal P wave axes due to ectopic atrial rhythms.

Certain cardiac operations are associated with particular rhythm disturbances. Transient sino-atrial and inter-atrial conduction disturbances are common after intra-atrial rerouting for transposition of the great arteries (Mustard operation) and repair of sinus venosus atrial septal defects. Simple secundum atrial septal defects also are associated with transient conduction abnormalities of this type.

Atrioventricular disturbances usually involve injury to the AV node itself or the common bundle of His. With present knowledge of the anatomy of the conduction system and facilities for intraoperative mapping, permanent heart block is uncommon after repair of uncomplicated ventricular septal defect, Tetralogy of Fallot and atrioventricular canal but temporary A–V dissociation is not uncommon particularly following the use of cold cardioplegia for myocardial preservation. Temporary pacing wires are necessary during the early postoperative hours. Right bundle branch block occurs following infundibular resection and right ventriculotomy. Usually the right bundle branch block is peripheral and of no prognostic significance, but if it is accompanied by left anterior hemiblock, complete heart block is a major hazard. His bundle conduction studies differentiate the left anterior hemiblock associated with the more ominous central right bundle branch block from the more benign peripheral variety. Injury, transient or permanent, of the left bundle branch may be anticipated following operations requiring incision or excision of portions of the ventricular septum.

Frequent premature ventricular contractions may be an indication of the severity of myocardial disease in patients with aortic stenosis or pulmonary hypertension. They are premonitory of sudden death and require aggressive treatment.

Temporary ventricular and atrial epicardial pacing wires are advisable after all open heart operations. Sequential (atrial and ventricular) pacing is useful for increasing the cardiac output, especially in patients with A–V dissociation, ventricular hypertrophy and poorly compliant ventricles: in these patients, having the atria and ventricles beat in proper synchrony may increase the cardiac output by up to 20%. Pacing thresholds are determined in the theatre and at least daily in any patient showing conduction abnormalities and requiring pacing. It is difficult to generalize as to which patients will require long-term, permanent pacing, but permanent pacemaker wires are best inserted at the end of the operation in all children with ventriculo-arterial discordance or with univentricular heart in whom even temporary A–V dissociation is observed during surgery.

If permanent pacing becomes necessary, the patient's small size is no deterrent, as techniques and equipment that are suitable for children have been developed.

5. Respiratory Problems

Most children may immediately resume spontaneous ventilation after uncomplicated cardiac operations such as patent ductus arteriosus, coarctation of the aorta, systemic pulmonary shunts, and intracardiac repair of uncomplicated atrial and ventricular septal defects. Most neonates and all infants and children having operations for more complicated cardiac problems than those listed above are best treated with at least a short period of ventilatory assistance.

An uncuffed nasal endotracheal tube is an easily secured and well tolerated means of maintaining airway patency. When an oral endotracheal tube has been used during surgery, it is replaced with a nasal tube at the completion of the operation unless a very short period of ventilatory support is anticipated. The size of the tube is such that it allows a small leak of air or gas around it with positive pressure ventilation. A tube slightly smaller than the one used during the operation allows room for the development of oedema, preventing prolonged subglottic irritation. The nasal tube protrudes no further than 10 mm from the alae nasae to prevent kinking and is securely positioned and fastened to the forehead as shown in Fig. 16.1. Following placement of the nasotracheal tube, a nasogastric tube is inserted to prevent gastric dilatation compromising respiration, and regurgitation and aspiration of gastric contents.

Immediately upon arrival in the intensive care unit, the child's endotracheal tube is connected to a volume cycled ventilator. Pressure cycled ventilators (e.g. Bird) are unsuitable for small patients. The inspired oxygen or gas is humidified and the tidal volume adjusted according to the volume used in theatre. The same applies to the oxygen concentration in the inspired gas mixture—usually ventilation in the intensive care unit is started with 80–100% F_1O_2 (page 111). Both tidal volume and F_1O_2 are then adjusted according to the results of the blood gas measurements (Pco_2, Po_2), which are measured at frequent intervals. The Po_2 is kept above 70 mmHg and the Pco_2 between 35–40 mmHg. The F_1O_2 can then be gradually reduced before the weaning process is started. Maintaining an adequate Po_2 may be assisted by providing positive end expiratory pressure (PEEP). PEEP of more than 10 cmH$_2$O tends to reduce systemic venous return and thus the cardiac output. Generally, the lowest level of PEEP is used that is shown to be effective.

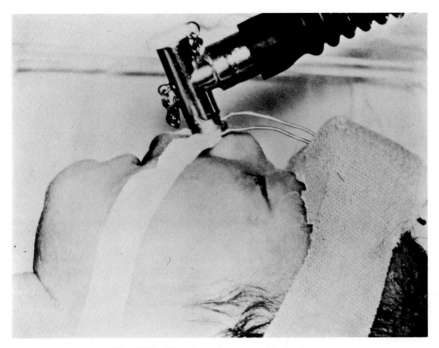

Fig. 16.1. Fixation of nasotracheal tube.

a. CARE OF PATIENTS ON VENTILATORS

All children with an endotracheal tube, whether ventilated or on the constant positive airway pressure (CPAP) system are sedated. In the first 24 hours, sedation with morphine sulphate is the most satisfactory. The first dose —i.v. or i.m.—is small, 0.1 mg/kg, because some children may be sensitive to morphine immediately after cardiopulmonary bypass. Subsequent doses are 0.2 mg/kg at 4 hourly intervals as required. Morphine can be supplemented with diazepam (valium) 0.1–0.3 mg/kg. It is important, however, to remember that diazepam lacks analgesic properties. If ventilatory support is required for several days or weeks, trichloral (30 mg/kg) usually provides adequate sedation.

b. PHYSIOTHERAPY

Pulmonary physiotherapy is an important part of respiratory care in infants and children. Secretions are aspirated from the nasal passages and oropharynx as required because children, particularly infants, do not swallow these secretions. The endotracheal tube's small size makes it liable to become obstructed by inspissated secretions; it is therefore frequently irrigated with small quantities of saline (0.5–1 ml in an infant) followed by catheter aspiration. The suction catheter is kinked, passed down the tube and suction applied only upon withdrawal. Continuous humidification of the inspired oxygen or gas mixture avoids inspissation of secretions, and frequent changes of position and chest percussion prevent pooling of secretions in the tracheobronchial tree. In infants, chest percussion is replaced by manual compression of the chest synchronous with ventilation. Mild hyperventilation with a hand bag before and during chest percussion is also useful. After extubation of infants, difficulties in removing secretions and recurrent episodes of atelectasis are treated by deep suction, accomplished by temporarily passing an endotracheal tube without anaesthesia, followed by saline irrigations, suction and mild hyperventilation using the hand bag. This procedure is effective and may be repeated several times daily.

c. WEANING FROM VENTILATORY SUPPORT

When the cardiovascular system is stable, weaning from the ventilator can be started. Other than primary pulmonary problems, relative contraindications to early weaning from mechanical assistance include a low cardiac output state, phrenic nerve paralysis in infants, generalized debilitation and central nervous dysfunction or seizures.

If PEEP has been used, it is first reduced and the F_1O_2 is then gradually reduced to 0.4–0.5. Providing the arterial Po_2 is maintained at 70 mmHg or more, and the arterial Pco_2 at 50 mmHg or less, the child will probably breathe spontaneously. These criteria do not, of course, apply to children with residual right-to-left shunts (for example, pulmonary atresia with VSD after aorto-pulmonary shunt operations).

The patient's endotracheal tube is disconnected from the ventilator and connected to a T-piece to provide oxygen and humidity, while allowing spontaneous ventilation. Alternatively the patient with the endotracheal tube in place but disconnected from the ventilator is placed directly into a humidified oxygen tent (child) or head-box (infant). If he is able to breathe spontaneously, but requires PEEP to maintain an adequate arterial Po_2, a constant positive airway pressure (CPAP) system is connected to the endotracheal tube, allowing the patient to regulate his own Pco_2, while providing assistance for arterial oxygenation. When the above manoeuvres do not allow the child to resume his own ventilation spontaneously, an intermittent mandatory ventilation (IMV) system may be used. The patient breathes spontaneously but is assisted with ventilations from the machine several times per minute. This will gradually allow separation from mechanical support. This method is particularly important for preventing diffuse atrophy of the respiratory muscles and for maintaining the child's cognizance of the stimulus to breathe.

Although most patients will resume adequate spontaneous ventilation in a day or so with one or more combinations of the above techniques, occasionally children will require weeks or even months. One must not be discouraged by these exceptions, since many initial failures finally become long-term successes. The techniques, which are similar to those used for adult patients, are applicable to even the smallest infants. Following removal of the endotracheal tube, stridor is occasionally present. This complication is managed with humidification using a tent, adequate sedation, dexamethasone 0.25 mg/kg i.v. and then 0.1 mg/kg i.v. for 3–4 doses. Prolonged nasal or oral endotracheal intubation with mechanical ventilatory support may be continued for days or weeks without the danger of subglottic stenosis.

Indications for tracheostomy are few. They include prolonged nasotracheal intubation when an adequate leak around the tube cannot be maintained, because there is then a danger of subglottic stenosis developing. Other indications are severe decubitus of alae nasi and thick secretions which may be more easily aspirated through a short tracheostomy tube. Tracheostomy also facilitates feeding and general handling of the infant and facilitates the weaning process. It can be performed safely even in the smallest infants, using the technique described by Aberdeen (1968).

Phrenic nerve paralysis is a major problem when it occurs postoperatively in infants. Infants normally are diaphragmatic breathers with the thoracic musculature being incompletely developed. Even unilateral phrenic nerve paralysis is tolerated poorly by infants and most require prolonged support. Infants appear to be especially vulnerable to the effects of phrenic nerve paralysis because their diaphragms are more mobile compared with those of adults and they are usually in the recumbent position which favours encroachment of the abdominal viscera upon the pleural space. Phrenic nerve paralysis may occur from direct trauma during any cardiac operation because of its proximity to the pericardium. Infants undergoing systemic-pulmonary shunt operations develop transient paralysis due to traction on the nerve. The paralysis may be masked while the patient is on positive pressure ventilation, because the diaphragm will not be elevated on chest x-ray and any infant who experiences difficulty in resuming spontaneous ventilation postoperatively should have fluoroscopic screening to determine whether paradoxical diaphragmatic movement is present. The diagnosis may also be suspected by an elevated arterial Po_2 with normal Po_2 when PEEP is withdrawn.

Following prolonged mechanical ventilation, even of months' duration, most patients will eventually be able to breathe spontaneously, although they may require tracheostomy as a weaning measure in the interim. Diaphragmatic plication may sometimes be necessary for intractable respiratory insufficiency due to phrenic nerve paralysis.

6. Fluid, Electrolyte and Metabolic Problems

Fluid balance may be critical in small infants. Based on the concept that fluid and sodium retention occurs after operation, fluids are best restricted to 5%

dextrose in water, giving 20 ml/m²/hour on the day of operation, 30 ml/m²/hour on the first postoperative day, and 40 ml/m²/hour the next day. This formula serves as a guide, with urinary output and measurements of serum and urinary chemistry allowing minor alterations. The best method of preventing water and electrolyte abnormalities is to start oral feeding, which is usually possible on the first day following operation.

a. WATER

When calculating fluid balance, *all* fluids given are recorded, i.e. intravenous fluids used for flushing arterial, atrial and venous lines, and anything given via a nasogastric tube. Under 'output', urine and nasogastric aspirate are recorded, with profuse diarrhoea or excessive sweating taken into consideration.

The criteria for fluid restriction are similar to those used in adults. Because of the danger of fluid overload in small infants, it is preferable to calculate the fluid administration per hour rather than for the whole 24 hour period. An error in fluid intake during one hour can easily be corrected in the next two or three hours. Ambient temperature and humidity are taken into consideration. This means that fluid intake may differ slightly during the winter and summer months.

If there are no signs of fluid retention, normal fluid intake is started on the third or fourth postoperative day. In most patients, however, a diet with no added salt is preferred for the first 3–4 weeks. Should the patient require antifailure treatment, such as digoxin and diuretics, moderate fluid restriction is continued for the first few weeks.

Diarrhoea may complicate the postoperative management of infants. Causes of diarrhoea include alteration of intestinal bacterial flora by antibiotics, pathogenic bacterial infections of the alimentary tract, lactose intolerance, and hypertonic milk formulas. Control of diarrhoea must be prompt to avoid fluid and electrolyte abnormalities. Oral feeding is stopped for 12–24 hours, giving the calculated fluid and electrolyte requirement intravenously. Usually diarrhoea abates in 12–24 hours. Eight to 12 hours after the diarrhoea has stopped, oral dextrose or salt solution is started followed by half strength, then full strength formula.

b. POTASSIUM

Potassium is added to the infusion, usually 3 mmol of potassium chloride in 100 ml of 5% dextrose. Should the serum potassium be below 3 mmol/l, the amount in the infusion may be increased to 3 mmol in 50 ml of 5% dextrose. Rapid administration of potassium is particularly hazardous in the small child. A simple calculation illustrates this point. For a 2.5 kg infant, the blood volume is 212 ml with the serum approximately 140 ml. Theoretically, the infusion of less than 0.3 mmol/l of potassium would raise the serum potassium concentration from 5 mmol/l to over 7 mmol/l. If the infusion takes place more rapidly than intracellular equilibrium of potassium can occur. Therefore, rapid potassium administration, or potential accidental rapid administration, cannot be tolerated.

c. SODIUM

Because the neonate's renal function is not mature, he excretes water loads less rapidly and conserves sodium less easily than adults. In these patients, it is necessary to be especially critical about the amount of water administered, giving small amounts of salt—one-tenth or one-fifth normal saline—with the intravenous fluids. Hyponatraemia, as in adults, is usually a manifestation of water overload but may occur due to salt depletion following long-term diuretic therapy. It is rarely necessary to treat dilutional hyponatraemia with more than fluid restriction.

d. CALCIUM AND MAGNESIUM

Low serum calcium and magnesium can cause problems postoperatively, particularly in neonates. Diuretics tend to deplete them also. These disorders are suspected when clinical signs of neuromuscular irritability appear and the diagnosis is confirmed by laboratory determinations. Hypocalcaemia is treated by giving 2–3 mmol calcium gluconate/kg/day intravenously or orally. Magnesium is given as 3% magnesium sulphate, 1 mmol/kg/day intravenously, intramuscularly or orally.

e. GLUCOSE

Neonatal hypoglycaemia may occur because hepatic glycogen stores are small. An initial infusion of 1–2 ml/kg of 50% dextrose followed by infusion of 10–15% dextrose in amounts equivalent to the patient's fluid regimen will usually control the hypoglycaemia.

f. OSMOLALITY

Hyperosmolality is a particularly devastating condition, causing cerebral oedema and intracerebral haemorrhage. Hyperosmolality and hypernatraemia often follow excessive administration of sodium, usually from overtreatment with sodium bicarbonate. Sodium bicarbonate (8.4%) has 2 mosmol/ml, 50% dextrose has 2.75 mosmol/ml, and 25% mannitol has 1.6 mosmol/ml. It should also be remembered that cardioconray used for angiocardiography has *1400* mosmol/ml. A guideline for preventing hyperosmolality is the administration of no more than 5–6 mosmol/kg/hour.

g. METABOLIC ACIDOSIS/ALKALOSIS

Postoperative metabolic *acidosis* is usually associated with a low cardiac output. Frequent determinations of arterial pH and base deficit will detect abnormalities before they become severe. The dose of sodium bicarbonate or THAM is calculated as: the base deficit in mmol/l × the body weight in kg × 0.3. To avoid overcorrection with resultant hypernatraemia and hyperosmolality, one half of the calculated dose is given and the blood gases repeated.

Using CPD rather than ACD blood during or after operation helps to avoid severe metabolic *alkalosis*. Nevertheless, it does occur, associated with potassium or chloride depletion, diarrhoea and infusions of large amounts of sodium bicarbonate. Metabolic alkalosis is treated by eliminating the underlying causes and by administering potassium chloride.

h. NUTRITION

The caloric requirement for normal growth of an infant is 100 kcal/kg/day but may be as high as 150 kcal/kg/day after operation. It is often difficult to provide these calorific requirements during the immediate postoperative period. Oral or nasogastric tube feeding is begun as soon as possible, which is usually 12 hours after operation. A nasogastric tube is kept in place so that any gastric residue can be aspirated and reflux with possible aspiration avoided.

The first feeding is with 5% dextrose in water. If tolerated, it is followed by half-strength milk or formula. Infants start oral or nasogastric feeding with a proportion of their hourly fluid requirement. The rest is used for flushing the indwelling catheters. When the feeds are well tolerated, the volume is increased and the interval between feeds is also increased to 2 or 3 hours.

The calorific intake can be increased by high calorie milk or medium chain triglycerides. If the child does not tolerate feeds for prolonged periods, intravenous alimentation is considered. This is also considered in patients who are in renal failure. Various regimes of intravenous hyperalimentation are recommended. They usually contain hypertonic glucose, amino-acids (Vamin) and lipids (Intralipid) (page 134).

7. Body Temperature

A major basal metabolic requirement and determinant of oxygen consumption for children is the maintenance of body temperature. Shivering increases oxygen demands also. Because homoeostatic mechanisms for maintaining body temperature are immature in small infants, there is a special tendency for them to develop hypothermia. Temperature is therefore closely monitored, keeping the ambient temperature at approximately 30°C and the patient's temperature as near 37°C as possible. Infra-red warmers are used for small children and infants.

Hyperthermia (pyrexia) demands investigation for sepsis. An elevated core (rectal) temperature associated with cool extremities suggests a low cardiac output state for which specific therapy is indicated as described earlier.

Like adults, children may develop pyrogenic reactions after open heart surgery. Rectal administration of aspirin, 15 mg/kg 4 hourly, tepid sponge baths and cooling blankets control modest temperature elevations. Markedly elevated temperatures (those above 40°C) require more aggressive treatment because of the elevated metabolic demands they impose. Sometimes refractory hyperthermia may require vasodilating agents, such as sodium nitroprusside or rogitine infusions, or largactil intravenous injections. Vasodilatation can also be achieved with high doses of steroids (Solumedrol 30 mg/kg/body weight, 6 hourly in 4–6 doses). Hyperpyrexia resistant to all these can be effectively controlled by peritoneal dialysis using a cooling coil.

8. Renal Problems

Management of postoperative renal failure follows the same principles as in adults (Chapter 10). Complete anuria suggests obstruction at some point in the urinary system, such as catheter obstruction, a congenital anomaly or renal vein thrombosis. Oliguria is defined as a urine volume of less than 0.5 ml/kg/hour. At the onset of such oliguria, the cardiac output is assessed as described in the cardiovascular section. If the cardiac output is low, an infusion of dopamine (2–5 µg/kg/min) or of isoprenaline (0.03–0.16 µg/kg/hour) is started. The catecholamines may increase the cardiac output and, in addition, dopamine may increase the renal perfusion. A diuretic is given—frusemide 1 mg/kg intravenously, increasing the dose to 3–5 mg/kg if there is no response at the lower doses. A test of mannitol (0.2 g/kg) or ethacrynic acid (1 mg/kg) may also be tried.

Hyperkalaemia complicating renal failure is treated with calcium resonium retention enemas, giving 1 g/kg and repeating hourly. Earlier use of peritoneal dialysis makes this regime rarely used. For life-threatening hyperkalaemia, 0.5 ml/kg of 10% calcium gluconate (0.11 mmol) is given, metabolic acidosis corrected if present and 1.5 g/kg of glucose plus one unit of insulin per 3 g of glucose infused.

PERITONEAL DIALYSIS

Peritoneal dialysis is begun early when diuretic-resistant anuria is present. Because the peritoneal surface of infants and children is larger, compared to body mass, than it is in adults, efficient peritoneal dialysis exchanges are possible.

In infants, the catheter is placed in the left flank, lateral to the rectus sheath. In older children, the optimal position is in the midline below the umbilicus, making sure that the bladder is empty at the time of insertion. The risk of visceral or major vessel injury is minimized by first injecting dialysis fluid into the abdomen via a small intravenous cannula. Aseptic technique during these procedures is essential.

The dialysis cycle is usually calculated at 30 ml/kg body weight. In some instances, this volume may cause respiratory embarrassment and may be reduced at least temporarily. A heating (cooling) coil is included in the circuit. Heparin (500 units/l) is added to the dialysate. Additional 50% dextrose is used to remove fluid from the patient more quickly if necessary. Once the child becomes normokalaemic, 4 mmol of KCl per litre is added. Antibiotics are added to the dialysate with a specimen of dialysate examined daily for cells and organisms prior to culture. Fluid balance is recorded carefully, because weighing the patient with his monitors and lines attached is logistically difficult. Nutrition is established as soon as possible to minimize catabolism. The detailed management of renal failure in infancy is well described by Chantler (1976) and Griffin *et al* (1976).

Occasionally, peritoneal dialysis may be used in the absence of renal failure to treat severe fluid overload, particularly in the presence of pulmonary oedema. It can be used, as stated above, to cool the hyperpyrexial infant.

9. Haematological Problems

Problems with postoperative bleeding, transfusions, haemolysis, coagulopathies, and long-term anticoagulation require special consideration by those caring for infants and children. The following scheme estimates blood volume in small patients: (1) for a body weight less than 10 kg, the blood volume is 85 ml/kg; (2) for a body weight of 10–20 kg, the blood volume is 80 ml/kg; and (3) for a body weight over 20 kg, the blood volume is 75 ml/kg.

One must realize that in an infant weighing 2 kg, a blood loss of 100 ml represents a loss of half its blood volume. Reoperation on a bleeding patient is recommended with a blood loss equivalent to 10% of blood volume in any one of the first three hours or a continuing loss equivalent to 5% of the blood volume per hour thereafter. Thus a loss of less than 20 ml per hour in the early postoperative hours may demand reoperation for haemorrhage (Table 16.5).

Similarly transfusions of small volumes are necessary. When anaemia with a haemoglobin of less than 10 g/100 ml is present, whole blood or packed red blood cells are transfused. The amount of blood necessary for transfusion is determined as follows: the percentage difference from normal of the patient's haemoglobin is multiplied by the calculated blood volume to estimate the total volume of the transfusion. The volume of packed red blood cells may be estimated to be 60% of whole blood, assuming the haemoglobin of bank blood to be 12 g/100 ml. Filters (40 micron) will prevent microemboli

Table 16.5. Suggested rules for reoperation for bleeding

Blood loss	1 yr	1–2 yr	2–4 yr	4–8 yr	8–16 yr	Approx. % of est. blood volume
ml in any 1 hour	70	85	130	180	350	10
ml/hour in any 2 consecutive hours	60	70	100	150	200	9
ml/hour in any 3 consecutive hours	45	55	80	110	210	6
ml total in 4 hours	150	175	250	350	700	20
ml total in 5 hours	175	200	300	450	850	25
Estimated blood volume	700	700–1000	1000–1600	1600–2000	2000–5000	100

and their use is recommended for all transfusions when the volume transfused approximates or exceeds one-half of the patient's blood volume. All blood is warmed before it is administered and in children in the early postoperative period 1 ml of 10% calcium chloride is given per 100 ml of CPD blood transfused to prevent myocardial depression.

A variety of coagulation abnormalities occur in polycythaemic children with cyanotic congenital heart disease. Preoperative erythropoiesis, replacing whole blood with plasma to obtain a haemoglobin below 20 g/100 ml, may ameliorate some of these bleeding problems. Although moderate degrees of thrombocytopenia are common after open heart operations, platelets are not given unless clinically important bleeding occurs and the platelet count is found to be less than 30 000/ml, when one unit of platelets is given for each 5 kg of body weight. Platelet counts lower than 20 000 may be associated with disseminated intravascular coagulation and sepsis. Fibrinolysis associated with clinically significant bleeding is treated by using epsilon aminocaproic acid (Cyklokapron 15 mg/kg slowly i.v., repeated 8 hourly if necessary). Excessive amounts of circulating heparin are neutralized by protamine (0.25 mg/kg) given slowly intravenously.

Postoperative haemoglobinuria due to haemolysis is treated with mannitol infusion (1 g/kg over 4–6 hours) to establish a urine flow of 5–10 ml/kg/hour. Sodium bicarbonate, 3 mmol/kg/hour, is then given to make the urine alkaline.

10. Jaundice

After cardiac operations jaundice may follow haemolysis, hepatitis, sepsis or bile duct obstruction and is managed as in adults (Chapter 12). Additional causes of obstructive jaundice in children include congenital anomalies of the biliary tract and calculi in patients with haemoglobinopathies. Physiological jaundice due to immature liver function in neonates appears after the first day of life and peaks during the first seven days. It seldom produces levels over 12 mg/100 ml (200 μmol/1) and is primarily indirect, unconjugated bilirubin. Neonatal jaundice is treated by phototherapy with exchange transfusion reserved for severe forms.

11. Infection

Infection is better prevented than cured as it causes a high mortality in infants especially. Complete prophylactic and therapeutic dental work including the removal or repair of all carious or deciduous teeth should be done prior to cardiac surgery.

The question of giving antibiotic cover before and during cardiac operations has not been universally resolved but the custom is to use antibiotics to cover both open and closed heart operations. Currently the antibiotic of choice is cloxacillin (12.5 mg/kg) every 6 hours for 3 days after closed operations, and for 5 days after operations involving cardiopulmonary bypass with the first dose being given four hours before operation. Children allergic to penicillin receive erythromycin (12.5 mg/kg 6 hourly). Both antibiotics are administered intravenously through the indwelling catheters. When the child restarts oral feeding, antibiotics are given orally. Neonates and young infants are more prone to infection caused by Gram-negative organisms and so, in addition to cloxacillin, all infants receive gentamicin (2 mg/kg 8 hourly iv./i.m.). Gentamicin is also given to older children who receive prosthetic valves, conduits and large prosthetic patches and to cover all reoperations.

Superficial monilial infections of the perineum and of the oral cavity (thrush) commonly occur in small children. At the first sign of monilial infection, Nystatin is used topically in the belief that suppressing this organism's presence on the child's cutaneous or mucous membranes will prevent systemic dissemination. In patients with thrush, Nystatin is also given orally (100 000 units 6 hourly).

Neonatal sepsis is the nemesis of all physicians treating paediatric patients. Signs and symptoms of neonatal sepsis include neurological manifestations (seizures, twitching, lethargy), cardiovascular changes, poor feeding, apnoeic episodes, jaundice, diarrhoea, hypothermia or hyperthermia. Often the only indication of sepsis is that the child is simply 'not doing well'. When specific symptoms or signs of sepsis appear, it may be too late to abort a fatal outcome; therefore, satisfactory treatment may require presumptive diagnosis only. In addition to the usual sites of postoperative infection in adults, the cerebrospinal fluid, umbilical stump and middle ear provide additional sources for sepsis. Prior to knowledge of the specific organism and antibiotic sensitivity, the child suspected of being septic is given both Gram-positive and Gram-negative coverage in high doses intravenously.

12. Neurological Problems

Unlike adults, children rarely have major psychological disturbances postoperatively; however, it would appear that psychological trauma is best avoided by performing operations before the age of 2 years or after the age of 4 years.

(a) *Neonatal seizures* are manifested by focal fits, or more usually, by generalized twitchings, in combination with apnoea and deviation of the eyes. Their diagnostic evaluation includes investigations for metabolic abnormalities, sepsis, intracranial haemorrhage, maternal diabetes and maternal narcotic addiction. Hypocalcaemia and/or hypoglycaemia are frequently the causes of fits in neonates. Hypocalcaemia may not be cured by calcium alone (1 mmol calcium/kg/day) and magnesium sulphate may be required in addition (0.25–0.5 mmol/kg/day). Diuretics in small babies may also cause fits due to hypocalcaemia. Hypoglycaemia is treated with intravenous glucose (1 ml/kg of 50% dextrose). If seizures are not controlled, diazepam (Valium) is given (0.1–0.5 mg/kg, i.v.). Chronic anticonvulsant therapy is started simultaneously, usually with phenobarbitone (1 mg/kg, 8–12 hourly).

(b) *Febrile seizures* associated with temperatures over 40°C occur in children during the first 3 or 4 weeks of life. When other causes have been ruled out, the temperature is lowered and diazepam or phenobarbitone given as above.

(c) *Ischaemic neurological disorders* are produced by cerebral air or particulate emboli, or by inadequate cerebral perfusion during or after cardiopulmonary bypass. Their manifestations include coma, flaccidity and seizures. Control of seizures is mandatory because they increase metabolic demands. Diazepam and phenobarbitone are given as above with dexamethasone (0.5 mg/kg, i.v. and then 6 hourly for 4–8 doses). Fluid restriction and mannitol infusions are useful additions.

13. Conclusions

Intensive care of infants and children with congenital heart defects should be aggressive. Special care techniques are used from the time of initial diagnostic suspicion, throughout the admission to the hospital, the diagnostic tests, the intraoperative period and during postoperative recovery and convalescence. It is only when the correct diagnosis is established early, the child operated upon before severe physiological and anatomical changes occur and the appropriate intensive care techniques used, that a reasonable survival rate is

Table 16.6. The Hospital for Sick Children, Great Ormond Street open heart surgery in the first year of life (1975–8)

Diagnosis	No.	Died	
		No.	(%)
Transposition of the great arteries + intact ventricular septum	49	3	6
Transposition of the great arteries × ventricular septal defect	16	5	31
Total anomalous pulmonary venous drainage	34	10	29
Ventricular septal defect	34	3	9
Persistent truncus arteriosus	20	13	65
Other	47	18	38
Total	200	52	26

achieved (Table 16.6). The current results of infant surgery have demonstrated a marked fall in mortality and morbidity over the last few years though there remain some lesions which still present a major challenge to all those caring for children with congenital heart defects.

REFERENCES

ABERDEEN E. (1968) Tracheostomy in infants. In *Operative Surgery* Vol. 2, 2nd edition. eds. C. Rob and R. Smith. Butterworths, London.

BAILEY L.L., TAKEUCHI Y., WILLIAMS W.G., TRUSLER G.A. & MUSTARD W.T. (1976) Surgical management of congenital cardiovascular anomalies with the use of profound hypothermia and circulatory arrest. Analysis of 180 consecutive cases. *J. thorac cardiovasc. Surg.* **71**, 485.

BARRATT-BOYES B.G., SIMPSON M. & NEUTZE J.M. (1971) Intracardiac surgery in neonates and infants using deep hypothermia with surface cooling and limited cardiopulmonary bypass. *Circulation suppl.* **43**, 25.

BRECKENRIDGE I.M., DIGERNESS S.B. & KIRKLIN J.W. (1970) Increased extracellular fluid after open intracardiac operation. *Surg. Gynec. Obstet.* **131**, 53.

CASTANEDA A.R., LAMBERTI J., SADE R.M., WILLIAMS R.G. & NADAS A.S. (1974) Open heart surgery during the first three months of life. *J. thorac. cardiovasc. Surg.* **68**, 719.

CHANTLER C. (1976) Management and prognosis of renal disease in childhood. Renal failure, urinary infections and hypertension. In *Recent Advances in Paediatrics* **5**, ed. D. Hull. Churchill Livingstone, Edinburgh.

COHN L.H., ANGELL W.W. & SHUMWAY N.E. (1971) Body fluid shifts after cardiopulmonary bypass. 1. Effects of congestive heart failure and hemodilution. *J. thorac. cardiovasc. Surg.* **62**, 423.

DE LEVAL M. & STARK J. (1974) Open heart surgery in the first year of life. *Acta Chir. Belg.* **73**, 481.

DUDRICK S.J. (1966) Total intravenous feeding and growth in puppies. *Fed. Proc.* **25**, 481.

ENGLISH T.A.H., DIGERNESS S. & KIRKLIN J.W. (1971) Changes in colloid osmotic pressure during and shortly after open intracardiac operation. *J. thorac. cardiovasc. Surg.* **61**, 338.

FILLER R.M., ERAKLIS A.J., ROBIN V.G. & DAS J.B. (1969) Long-term total parenteral nutrition in infants. *New Eng. J. Med.* **281**, 589.

FINBERG L. (1967) Dangers to infants caused by changes in osmolal concentration. *Pediatrics* **40**, 1031.

GREGORY G.A., KITTERMAN J.A., PHIBBS R.H., TOOLEY W.H. & HAMILTON W.K. (1971) Treatment of the idiopathic respiratory-distress syndrome with continuous positive airway pressure. *New Eng. J. Med.* **284**, 1333.

GRIFFIN N.K., McELNEA J. & BARRATT T.M. (1976) Acute renal failure in early life. *Arch. Dis. Childhood* **51**, 459.

HARRIES J.T. Aspects of intravenous feeding in childhood. In *Proceedings of an International Symposium held in Bermuda*, May 1977, ed. Ivan D.A. Johnston, Lancaster.

JORDAN S.C. & SCOTT O. (1973) *Heart Disease in Paediatrics.* Butterworths, London.

NADAS A.S. & FYLER D.C. (1972) *Paediatric Cardiology.* p. 665. W.B. Saunders, Philadelphia. [see Table 16.1].

PACIFICO A.D., DIGERNESS S. & KIRKLIN J.W. (1970) Acute alterations of body composition after open intracardiac operations. *Circulation* **41**, 331.

POOLEY R.W., HAYES C.J., EDIE R.N., GERSONY W.M. & BOWMAN F.O. (1976) Open heart experience in infants using normothermia and deep hypothermia. *Ann. thorac. Surg.* **22**, 415.

RUDOLPH A.M. & CAYLER G.C. (1958) Cardiac catherization in infants and children. *Pediat. Clin. N. Amer.* **5**, 907.

STARK J. (1978) Intensive care after intracardiac operations in infancy. In *Paediatric Cardiology* eds. R.H. Anderson & E.A. Shinebourne. Churchill Livingstone, Edinburgh.

STARK J., DE LEVAL M., MACARTNEY F. & TAYLOR J.F.N. (1980) Open heart surgery in the first year of life. Current state and future trends. In *Advances in Cardiology.* Karger, Basel.

ZEIGLER R.F. (1951) *Electrocardiographic Studies in Normal Infants and Children.* Charles C. Thomas. Springfield, Illinois. [see Table 16.2].

Index